"I love fashion. I love when people put me in it. And, God knows, I'm slowly getting better at putting stuff together myself."

−JENNIFER ANISTON

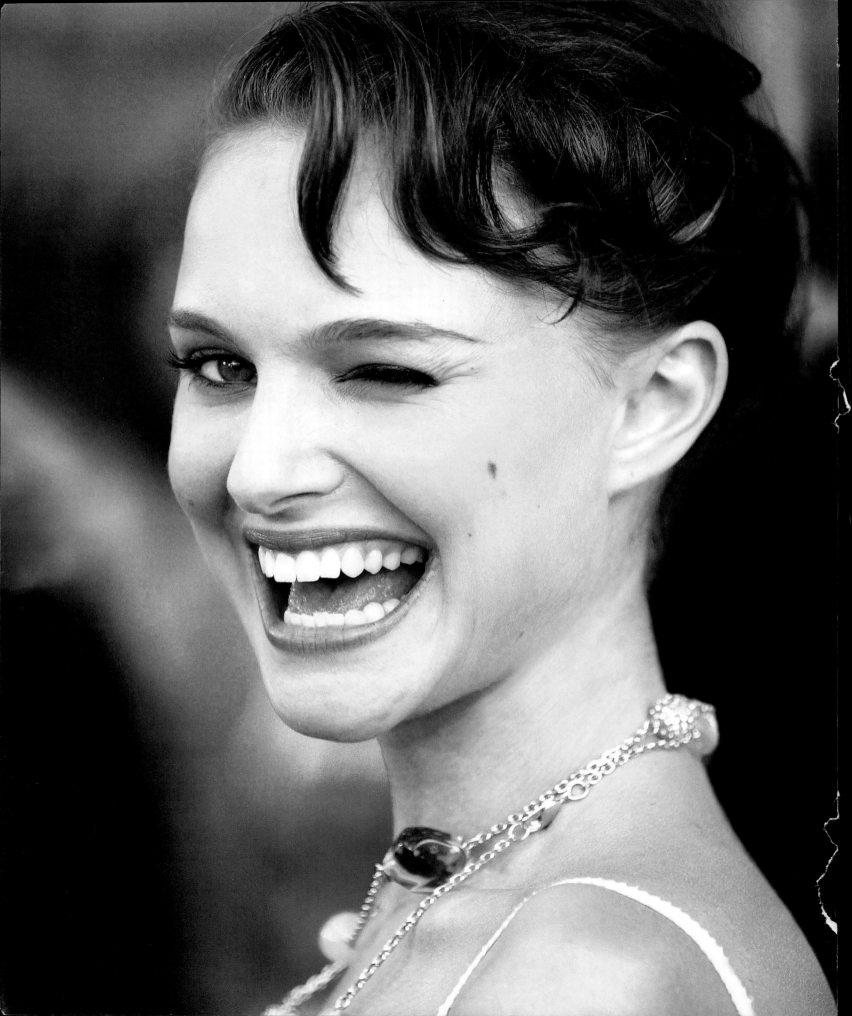

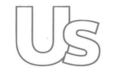

# SECRETS OF
# Celebrity
# Style

## A CRASH COURSE IN DRESSING LIKE THE STARS

FROM THE EDITORS OF *Us Weekly*

## WRITTEN BY DALE HRABI

DESIGN BY dk Design Partners Inc, NYC

WENNER BOOKS

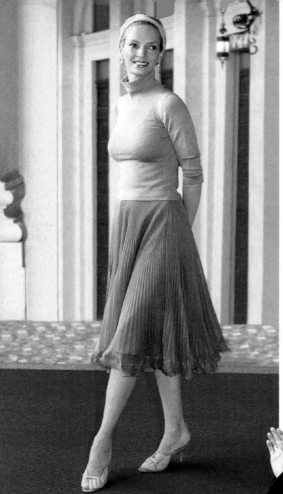

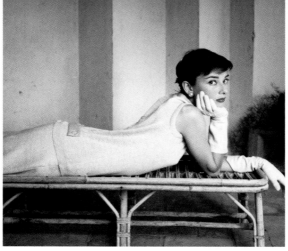

# CONTENTS

## part one

**TIMELESS**

The Look of Celebrity Style

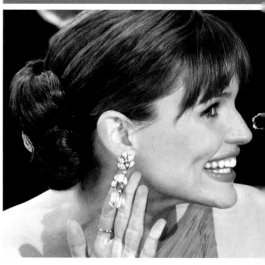

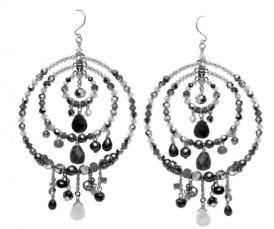

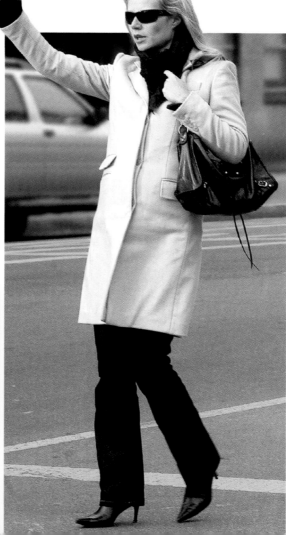

## part two

**STAR STYLE**

Five Ways to Make It Yours

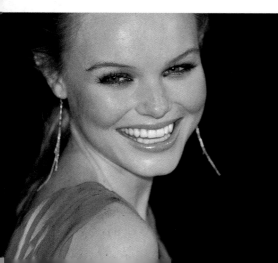

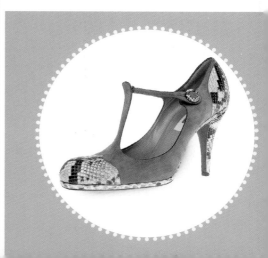

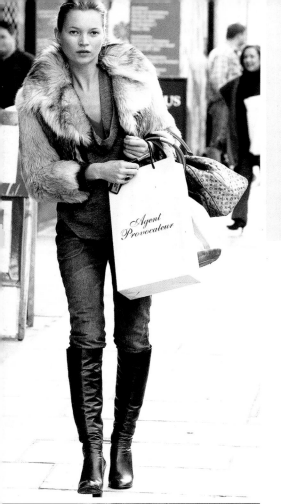

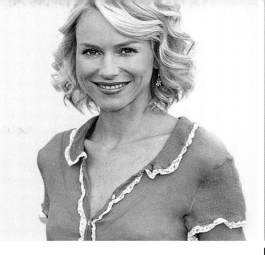

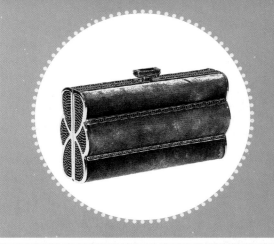

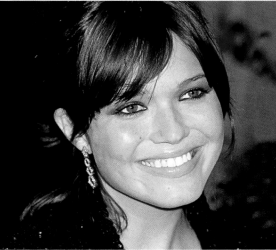

# part three

## OCCASIONS

Living with Celebrity Style

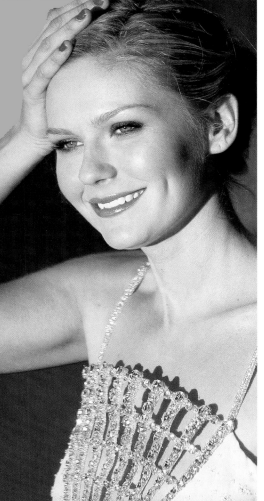

# part four

## STRATEGIES

Thinking Like a Celebrity Stylist

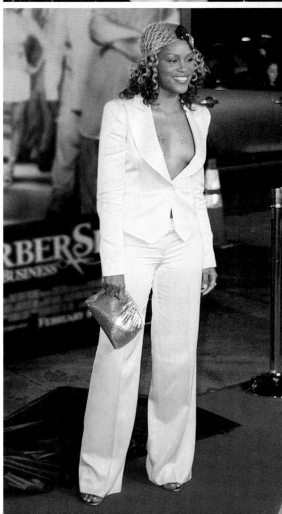

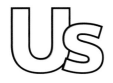

# SECRETS OF CELEBRITY STYLE

**Editorial Director** Dale Hrabi

**Contributing Creative Director** Kurt Houser

**Photography Director** Lisbet Oley

**Photo Editors** Caroline Sturgess, Jennifer Loeber

**Style and Accessories Editor** Ernestine Jean Lee

**Copy Editor** Robert Firpo-Cappiello

**Editorial Assistants** Carol McColgin, Kate Rockland

## ACKNOWLEDGEMENTS

**Many thanks to:**

Alysia Abbott, Elizabeth Betts, Lauren Bhatia, Debra Cardona, Daryl Chen,
Jen Daniels, Hannah Deely, Dina Dell'Arciprete, John Dragonetti, Cindy Evans,
John Gibson, Lynn Harris, Hayley Hill, Erin Hirsh, Karen J., Suzanne Marchese,
Paul Margolis, Pauline O'Connor, Laura Ogar, Jessica Pastor, Michael Pirrocco,
Linda Pitt, Miranda Purves, Jennifer Rade, Tamara Rappa, Tracey Reese,
Sara Rogers, Rachel Zoe Rosenzweig, Michael Skinner, Danielle Stella-Fischer,
Mary Alice Stephenson, Brittain Stone, Jill Swid, Robert B. Wallace, Danna Weiss

Please turn to page 218 for photo credits

Library of Congress Cataloging-in-Publication Data
Hrabi, Dale.
Us secrets of celebrity style : a crash course in dressing like the stars / Dale Hrabi.
p. cm.
Includes bibliographical references and index.

ISBN 1-932958-51-7

1. Women's clothing. 2. Celebrities–Clothing. 3. Motion picture actors and actresses–Clothing. I. Title.
GT1720.H73 2005
391'.2--dc22

2004026470

Wenner Books are available for special promotions and premiums. For details contact Michael Rentas, Manager, Inventory and Premium Sales, Hyperion, 77 West 66th Street, 11th floor, New York, New York 10023, or call 212-456-0133.

FIRST EDITION    10  9  8  7  6  5  4  3  2  1

I loved fashion growing up, but I never loved fashion magazines. The models were all so blank-faced, with no detectible personality, not to mention impossibly skinny and way too tall. Trying to imagine myself, at 5'2", wearing the same clothes seemed a waste of time. When I was in college in the early '90s, however, something happened: Hollywood began to rediscover old-school glamour in a big way and the stars started working the red carpet year round, not just at the Academy Awards. For me, that's when fashion got a lot more real. Like the rest of us, celebrities were all different shapes, some even as short as I was. They were obviously alive, and, because I'd seen their movies and TV shows, I felt as if I knew these women a little. The best part was when they talked about why they loved a dress, how hard it was to find the right one, or laughed at their more dubious style choices.

At *Us Weekly* magazine, our goal has always been to celebrate celebrity fashion at its most inspiring, but also to bring it down to earth. This book is designed to help you take the next step, to show you how to incorporate star style into your wardrobe at any age, no matter what you're shaped like, and for all kinds of occasions—from a simple shopping trip to a black-tie gala. And also to remind you that even stars (as they'll admit) don't always get it right, which allows us to learn from their mistakes and even to laugh at our own. Style, after all, should never be some uptight exercise in looking perfect. At its best, it's both glamorous and real, and never boring.

**Janice Min**, Editor-in-Chief, *Us Weekly*

# PART ONE

# TIME

## The Look

# A red dress that can stop hearts

might sound highly irresponsible, but—along with trench coats, sunglasses, and a well-aimed leopard spot or two—it's been part of the uniform of fame for 60 years. These are the sort of timeless elements that once made people stare at Audrey Hepburn or Marilyn Monroe and wonder: "Who is she?" Or that make us look at today's stars and think, half-seriously, "I want to be her." While *becoming* her would be excessive (how many Gwen Stefanis can one world handle?), who says you can't borrow the best parts of her look?

# LESS of Celebrity

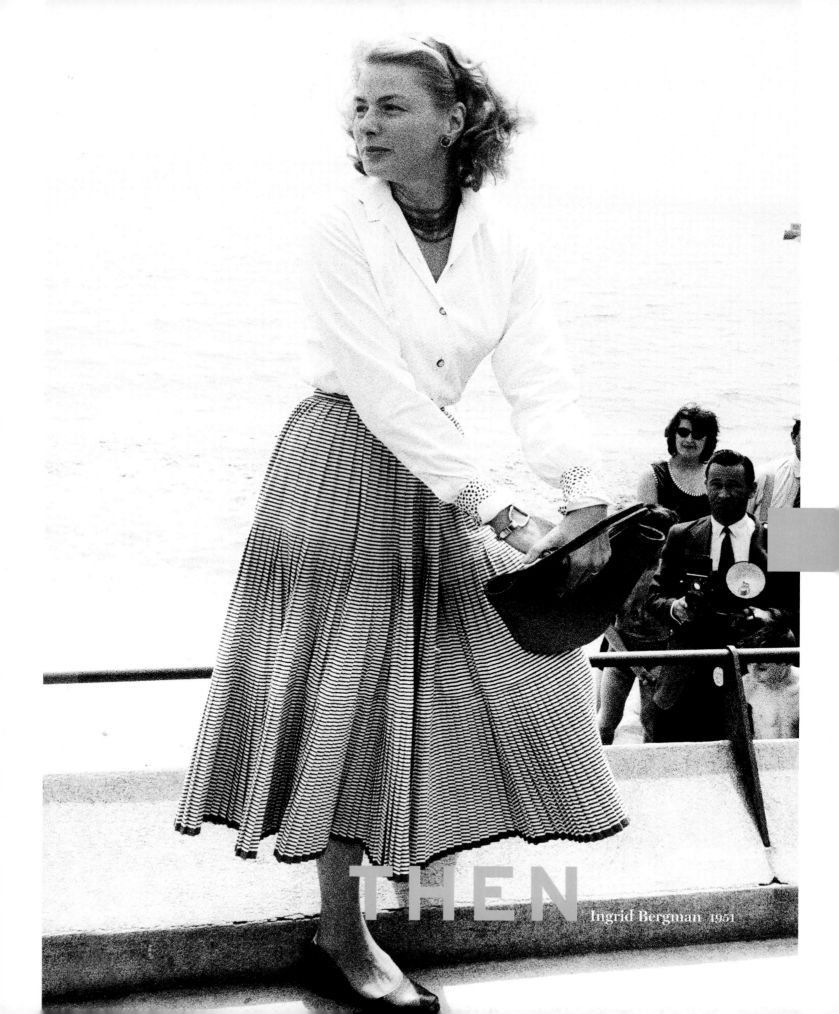

THEN

Ingrid Bergman 1951

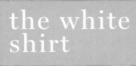

## the white shirt

It can give anyone star quality: The whiteness frames a face the way a theater's darkness frames a close-up.

**Mary J. Blige** **NOW**

# the little black dress

**Audrey Hepburn 1961**

**The L.B.D.** is the official dress of nonchalance, a perfect mix of "Look at me" and "oh, this little thing?" Variations on its small black formula are endless, but the ground rules haven't changed since Audrey Hepburn invested it with Hollywood glamour in 1961's *Breakfast at Tiffany's*. The shape should be simple with no more than a single flourish. A bow, a feathery hem, an all-that-glitters bag. Utterly elegant—yet no big deal.

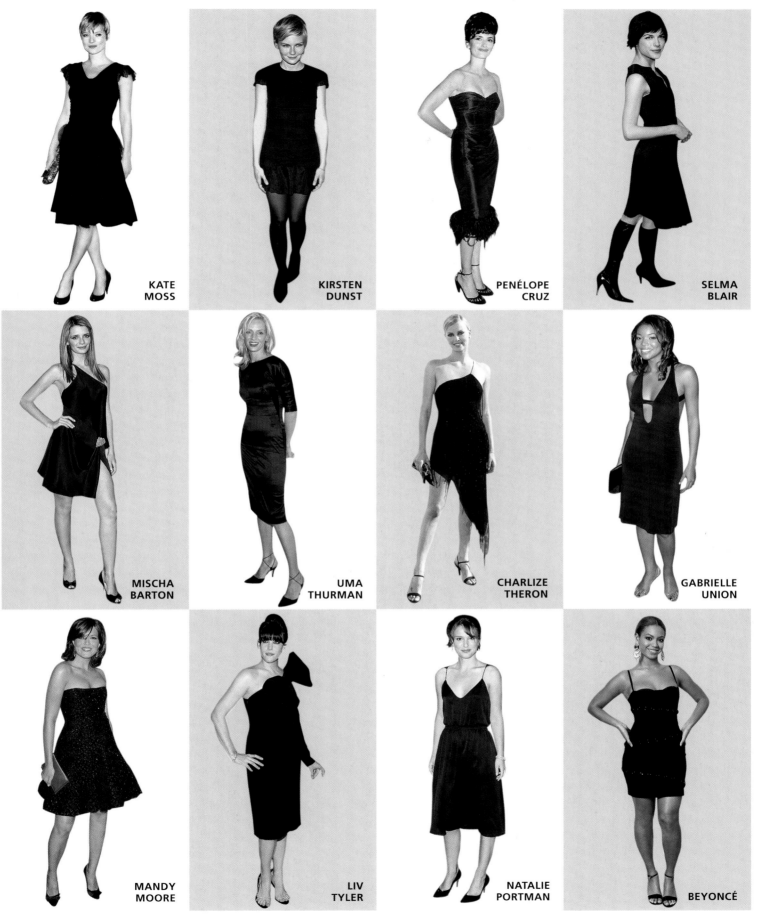

KATE
MOSS

KIRSTEN
DUNST

PENÉLOPE
CRUZ

SELMA
BLAIR

MISCHA
BARTON

UMA
THURMAN

CHARLIZE
THERON

GABRIELLE
UNION

MANDY
MOORE

LIV
TYLER

NATALIE
PORTMAN

BEYONCÉ

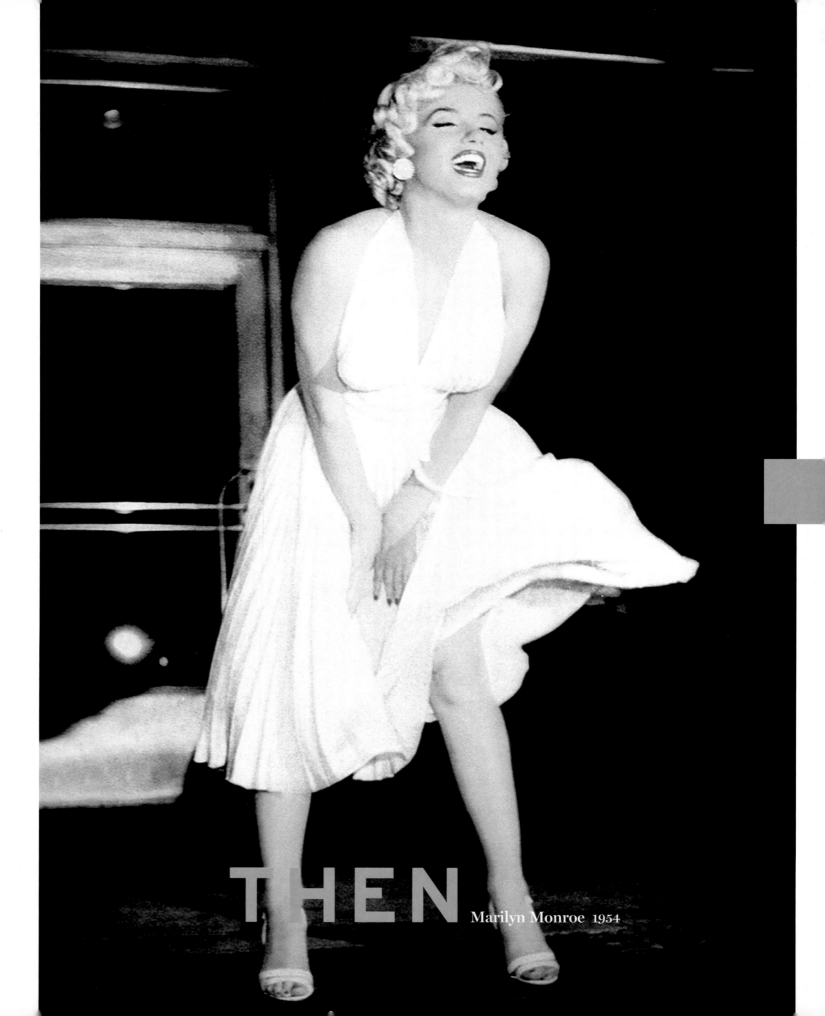

THEN Marilyn Monroe 1954

## the halter dress

Two eras. Two interpretations. Two completely different attitudes. One result: goddess.

Jessica Alba **NOW**

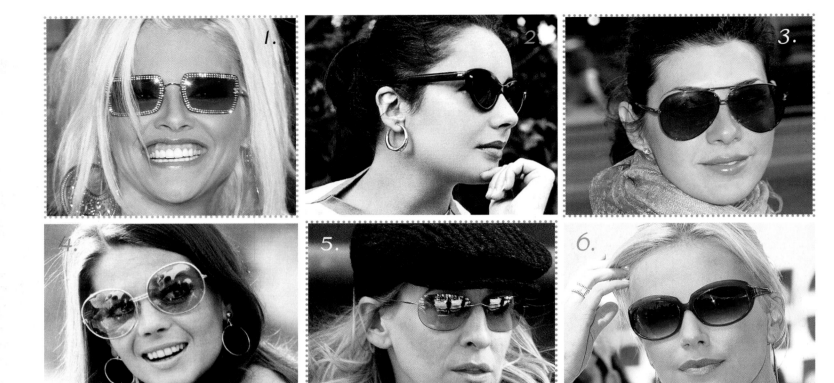

1.

2.

3.

4.

5.

6.

# Shades

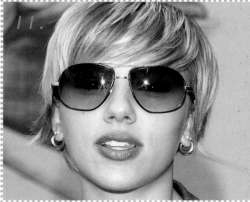

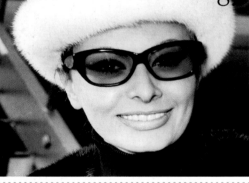

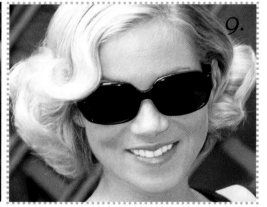

7.

8.

9.

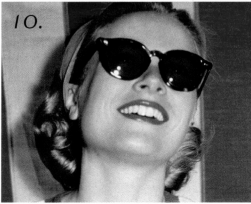

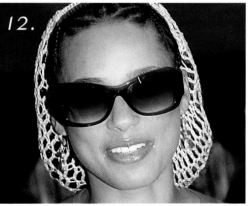

10.

11.

12.

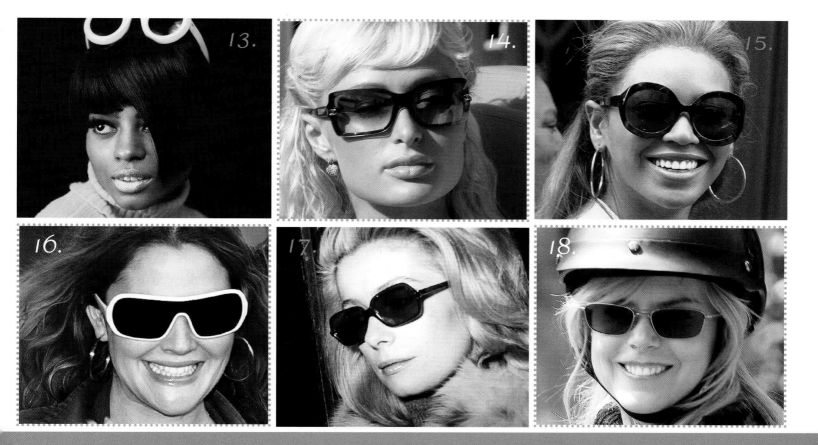

**Guess who?** A modern take on the veil, sunglasses are an intrigue strategy—and the best shortcut to glamour. Can you identify these enigmatic stars? (See page 220 for answers.)

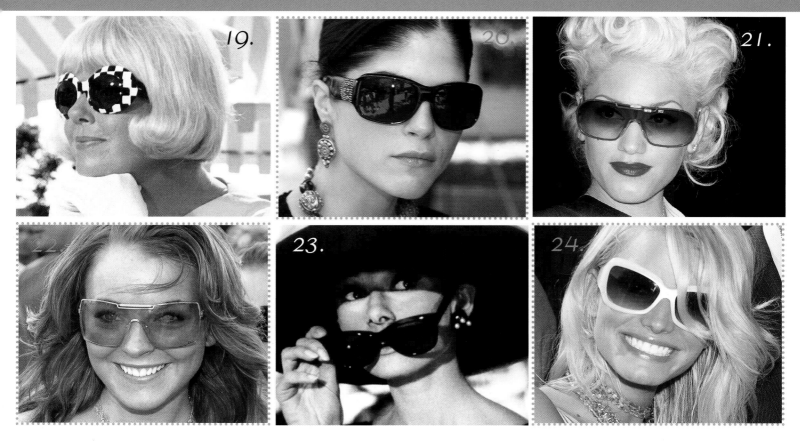

THEN Jacqueline Kennedy 1962

## the scarf

It has always been a key accessory in the uniform of fame, as a full-on diva flourish— or as a place to hide.

Jessica Simpson NOW

# THE SEXY RED DRESS

Whatever the vintage, the message is the same: Fire when ready…

## THE *Fifties*

Wasp-waisted with a full skirt, the '50s version is respectably wanton.

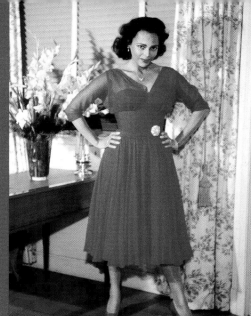

DOROTHY DANDRIDGE **1955**

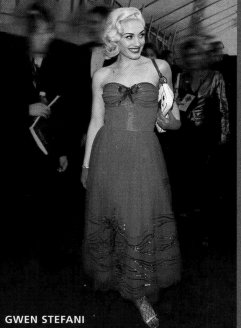

GWEN STEFANI

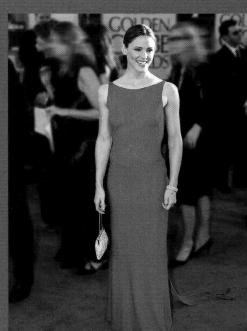

JENNIFER GARNER

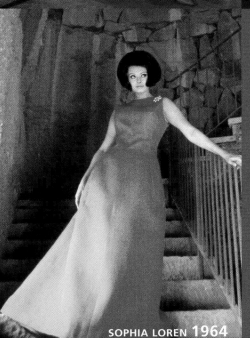

SOPHIA LOREN **1964**

## THE *Sixties*

Simpler, stronger, too modern to be coy, the '60s-inspired red dress doesn't fool around.

## THE *Seventies*

Hot went haute again with the first stirrings of the vintage glamour revival that rules today.

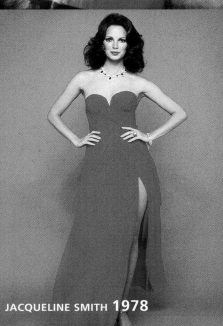

JACQUELINE SMITH **1978**

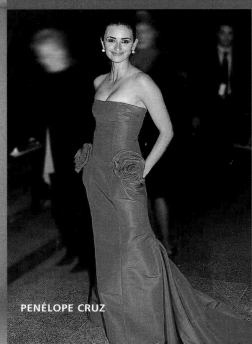

PENÉLOPE CRUZ

THEN

Zsa Zsa Gabor 1968

## the hot spot

It's the biggest Hollywood cliché, but leopard still bites right if it's worn sanely, as a single shot of wildness. A coat, a bag, or a pair of shoes. (Never all three.)

Kate Moss **NOW**

"Youth must be replaced with mystery," Coco Chanel once said. And when that time comes, get a trench coat. (Stars start early.)

TRENCHCOATS

Mia Farrow 1967

# Modern

The technicolor trench:
a traditionally quiet coat
expresses itself.

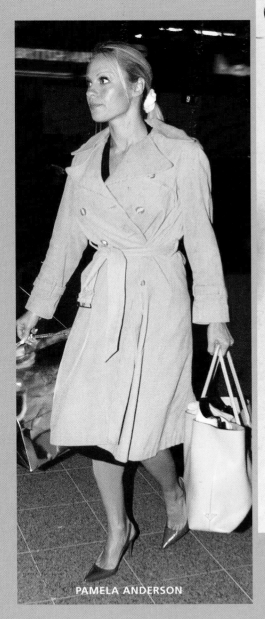

PAMELA ANDERSON

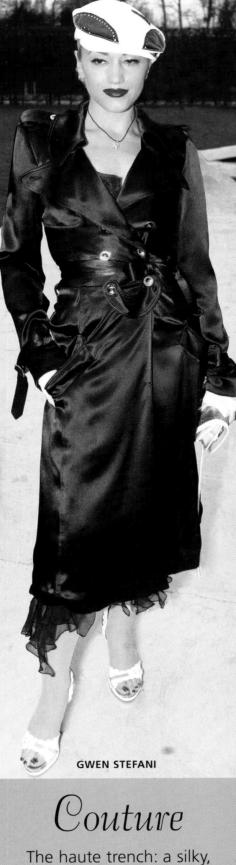

GWEN STEFANI

# Classic

The old-school British
trench: buttoned-up
and ready to spy.

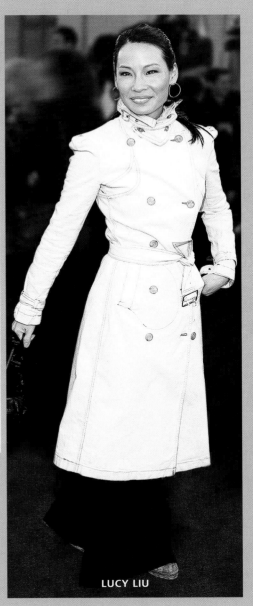

LUCY LIU

# Couture

The haute trench: a silky,
slinky revamp that's in no
way water-resistant.

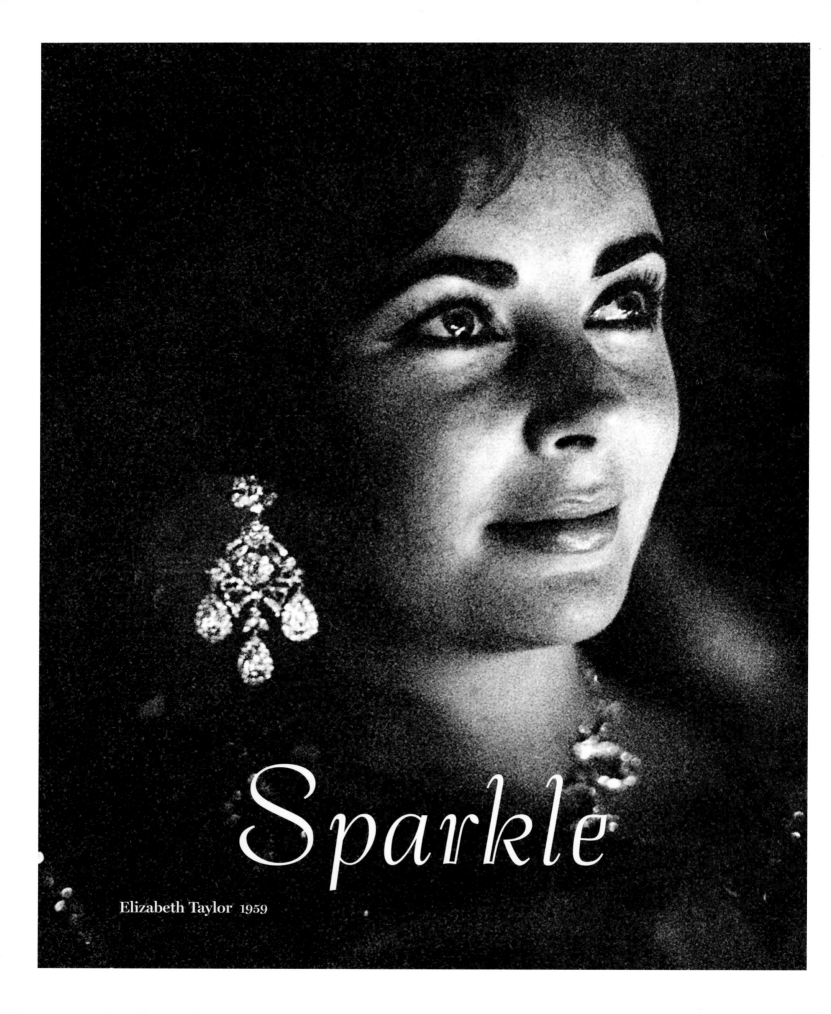

Sparkle

Elizabeth Taylor 1959

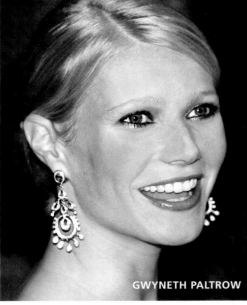

GWYNETH PALTROW

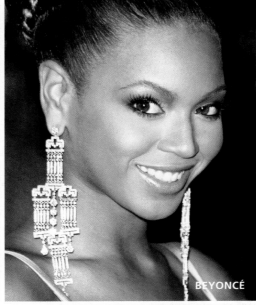

BEYONCÉ

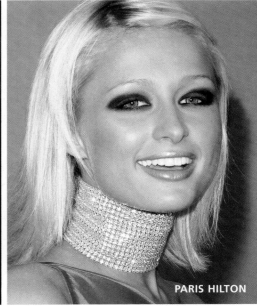

PARIS HILTON

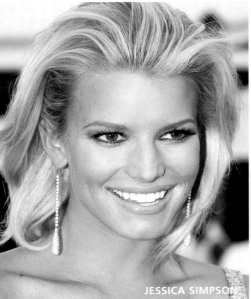

JESSICA SIMPSON

It's part of the job description: Stars, by definition, need to shine. Whether discreetly in a pair of silvery slingbacks, or unmistakably in that perennial favorite —*big rocks.*

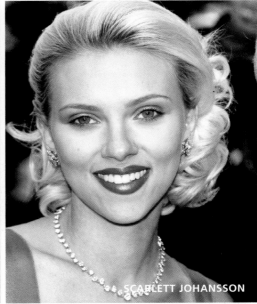

SCARLETT JOHANSSON

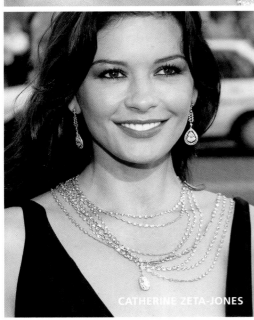

CATHERINE ZETA-JONES

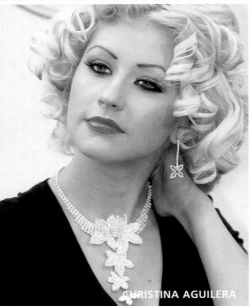

CHRISTINA AGUILERA

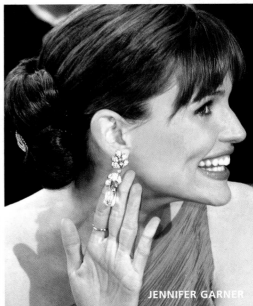

JENNIFER GARNER

THEN
Audrey Hepburn in Givenchy 1954

It takes guts to pull off gowns like these—both delicate and flamboyant. But wouldn't it be cruel to own such a beautiful thing, and never let it leave your closet?

## the showstopper

# NOW

Penelope Cruz pays homage in Oscar de la Renta

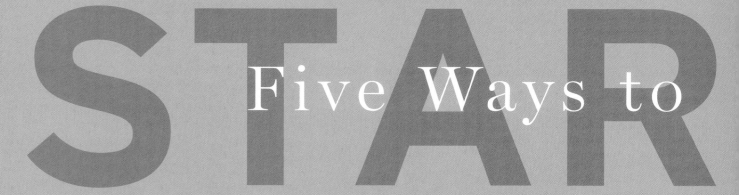

# PART TWO

Five Ways to STAR

# It takes more than a random

Valentino gown or a pair of sunglasses, of course, to nail star-caliber style. You need an overall strategy, one that edges up your glam factor but still connects with the deepest you (the you who hates ironing, or has a slightly uncool obsession with turtlenecks). To help you zero in on the right approach, and see how it all comes together, we've classified the stars into five style categories, from the classic elegance of **Renée Zellweger** to the eclectic chic of **Kirsten Dunst.** Which one's for you?

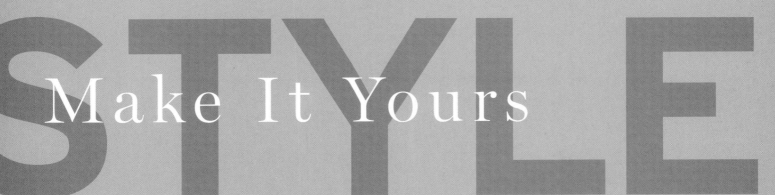

STYLE
Make It Yours

chapter *2*

# CLASSIC

Classic style is about keeping it simple. Not dull simple, or lonely nun simple. *Startlingly* simple and 100-percent guaranteed chic. It's for women—like **Nicole Kidman** or **Renée Zellweger** —who don't waste time making mistakes. Who like the

decisiveness of black, the clarity of white. Who prefer pounding rain to

drizzle. (Drizzle annoys them. It's too…wishy-washy.) If this look ultimately

works for you, it's likely you already avoid style clutter. You aren't opposed

to a ruffle with *purpose*, but feel that most frills lack a point. Ditto fringe…and

prints. (You'd make a terrible hippie.) You don't buy clothes on a whim any

more than you'd get married in a Vegas chapel. Or name your baby Puma.

You want pure elegance—the sort that occasionally makes jaws drop.

"Simplicity is the keynote
of all true elegance."

—COCO CHANEL

# Nicole Kidman

She once had a weakness for *Little House on the Prairie* pinafores. But over the years Nicole has pared her look back to a cool, **tailored minimalism.**

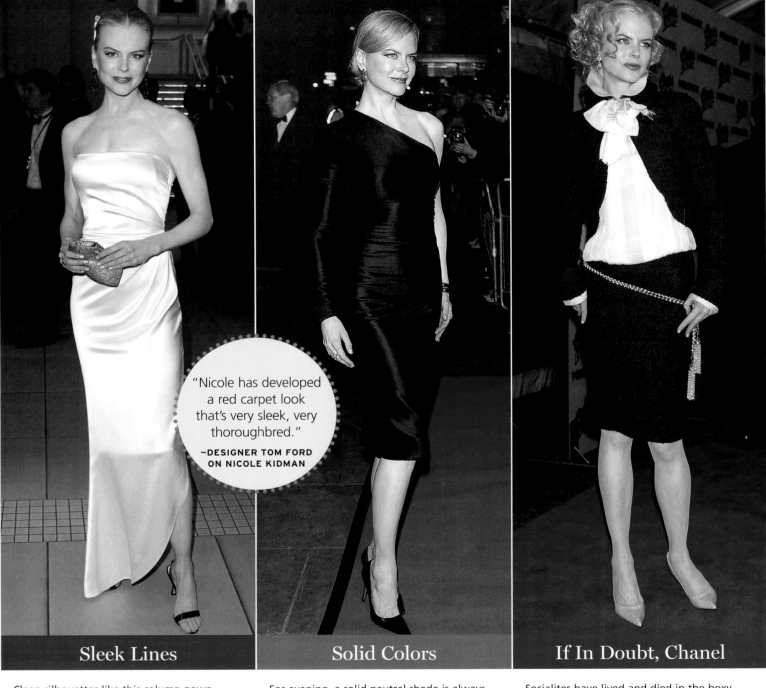

"Nicole has developed a red carpet look that's very sleek, very thoroughbred."

**—DESIGNER TOM FORD ON NICOLE KIDMAN**

## Sleek Lines

## Solid Colors

## If In Doubt, Chanel

Clean silhouettes like this column gown define classic. This cut can look stiff, but Nicole's vintage Ungaro, slit to the thigh, is fitted to skim her body, not mummify it.

For evening, a solid neutral shade is always more classic than a pattern. With its absentee sleeve, Nicole's asymmetrical sheath is a bit bratty, but its utter blackness keeps it classic.

Socialites have lived and died in the boxy, old-school Chanel suits, but Nicole, who never lets herself get locked in style prison, keeps it flirty in this 2003 version.

# Renée Zellweger

One of Hollywood's most consistently glam stars, she's long been a disciple of **circa-1960 restraint**. Swingy, loose hair helps her keep it modern.

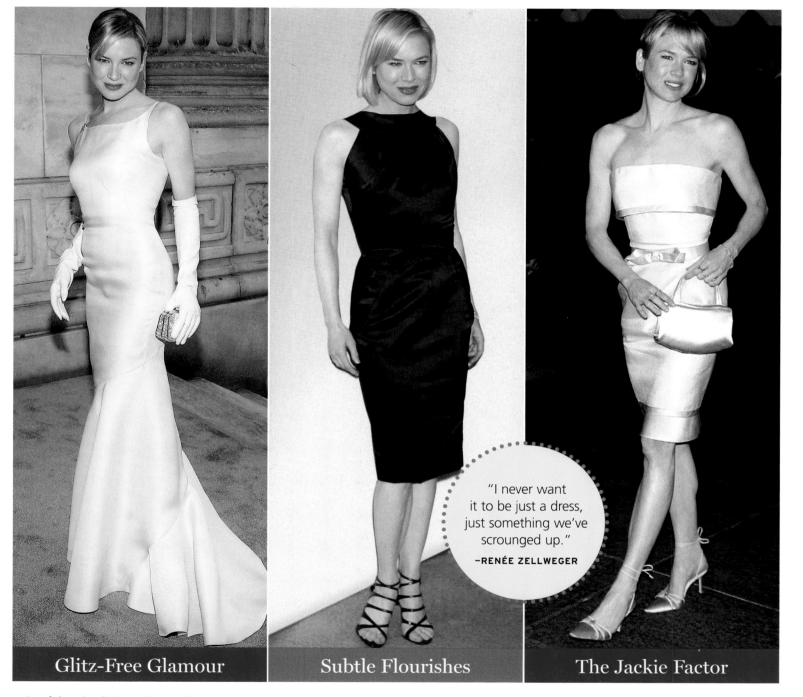

"I never want it to be just a dress, just something we've scrounged up."
—RENÉE ZELLWEGER

## Glitz-Free Glamour

Proof that simplicity can be regal: A basic sheath blossoms into a Carolina Herrera gown. No beading, it's all about shape. (Not suitable for work, unless you rule Spain.)

## Subtle Flourishes

A waistline bow peeks out of murky black on this distinctive vintage dress, from Lily et Cie in Los Angeles. Not so subtle: those dominatrix sandals. (What do you think...stupid or sexy?)

## The Jackie Factor

Channeling Jackie Kennedy in a 1962 Oleg Cassini dress. A classic strapless cut works best if you're a bit bustier than Renée here, but the extra satin fold makes it flattering.

# Natalie Portman

Insanely beautiful in the Audrey Hepburn mode, she's still experimenting with style, but often gravitates toward clean, **preppie-classic looks**.

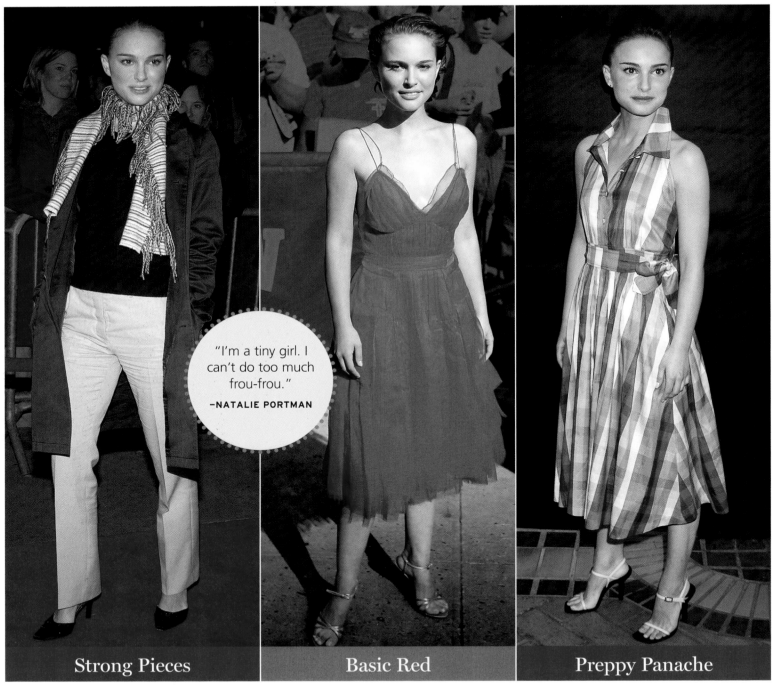

> "I'm a tiny girl. I can't do too much frou-frou."
>
> —NATALIE PORTMAN

### Strong Pieces

### Basic Red

### Preppy Panache

Use solid-color elements, like these pink Helmut Lang flat-fronts, as building blocks. True purists ban all pattern, but Natalie loops on a kitten-friendly striped scarf.

Too brassy to be classic? If the cut is straight-forward enough, red can be powerfully per-fect. Natalie softens her attack in an A-line Marc Jacobs dress in pleated chiffon.

Otherwise restrained, preppies sometimes wear loud prints in a "what the hell, we're rich" spirit. Natalie plays the game more ele-gantly in an Isaac Mizrahi halter dress.

# [**CLASSIC:** with a twist]

*Sexy design tweaks (and a little makeup anarchy) can give basic shapes a modern spirit, as Hollywood's young style virtuosos know.*

*Boyish haircut* ·····

*Punky orange eye-shadow*

*Unexpected color*

### Katie Holmes ➤
**in NARCISO RODRIGUEZ**
A little black dress gets a little bit rocker. Katie looks sweet with '60s ingenue hair and junior-league Prada pumps, but the dress's silver insets spike her look with bad-girl edge.

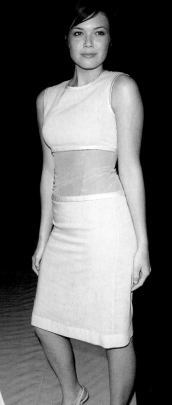

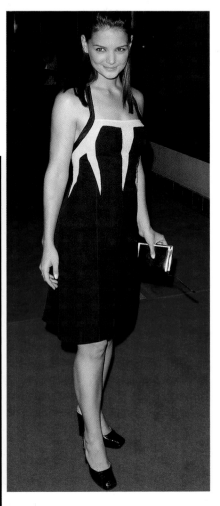

### ◀ Mandy Moore
**in NARCISO RODRIGUEZ**
A sheer-look midriff panel makes Mandy's cotton-and-voile version of the classic sheath dress politely *hot*. She ups the bareness factor by wearing no jewelry at all.

### ◀ Selma Blair **in BEHNAZ SARAFPOUR**
What makes this tulle-and-brocade vintage-inspired formal look so millennial? A waist ribbon that's bright yellow (instead of '50s white), plus antiprom makeup and hair.

# AUDREY HEPBURN

Patron Saint of Style

**i**t's ironic to call Audrey Hepburn's 1950s style "classic." At the time, she was a complete fashion radical. The prevailing glamour ideal was bosomy, wobbly, and tight—bulging sweaters and enfeebling stilettos. But in movies like *Sabrina* and *Breakfast at Tiffany's*, Audrey created a new model: streamlined, more subtly sexy, and actually mobile. A former ballet dancer with a formidable will (in her native Holland she survived a winter of Nazi deprivation by eating tulip bulbs), she had no use for predictable male fantasies of what "girls" should look like. She dressed for her own unbusomy body, dispensing with the whole idea of cleavage and unveiling other erogynous zones (shoulders! clavicles!) strategically. Women everywhere worshiped her defiance; in her little boat-

## Flats

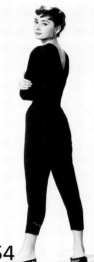

1954
AUDREY HEPBURN

2004
NATALIE PORTMAN

necked black dresses, white shirts, and slim black trousers—inevitably designed by her favorite couturier, Hubert de Givenchy—she defined what famed shoe designer Manolo Blahnik has called "the most important look of the 20th Century."

That look has always been grounded in versatile basics and accessories. In her book *Audrey Style*, Pamela Keogh quotes a dancer who worked with Hepburn during her late-1940s stint as a cash-starved London chorus girl: "[She seemed to own] one skirt, one blouse, one pair of shoes, and a beret, but she had 14 scarves. What she did with them week by week you wouldn't believe."

## Stripes

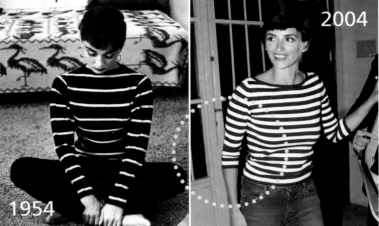

1954
AUDREY HEPBURN

2004

PENÉLOPE CRUZ

......................... **Nautical Stripes** .........................

**Then:** Audrey's stripes, as strong and direct as she was, can be traced to Chanel, who swiped the motif from French sailors in the 1930s.
**Now:** Decades later, Penelope Cruz traces the Hepburn lineage.

......................... **Ballet Flats** .........................

**Then:** Descended from Dutch aristocracy, young Edda Kathleen van Heemstra Hepburn-Ruston first called herself "Audrey" while studying ballet. She kept the name—and these graceful, much-copied flats.
**Now:** Natalie Portman pays heel-less homage.

......................... **Ribbon Bows** .........................

**Then:** This sweetly limp, unfussy bow was the sort of feminine detail Audrey used to humanize her stark black-and-white look.
**Now:** In a scene from *Sex and the City*, Kristin Davis (more predictably) ties one on pink.

## Bows

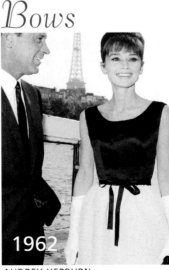
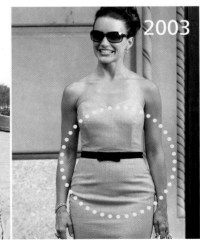

1962
AUDREY HEPBURN

2003

KRISTIN DAVIS

# get the look

Anyone can get hooked on classic. All it takes is a willingness to follow a formula—and the instinct to (occasionally) tweak that formula so it's right for you.

**Classic style may seem uncomplicated**—black plus simple equals bingo—but to really pull it off, it helps to be as ruthless as a dingo. As Coco Chanel said, "Elegance is refusal." That means saying no to anything too obvious. No to glitz, yes to sheen. No to cleavage, yes to glimpses. It's about learning to see the beauty in unadorned, tailored clothes and rejecting any trend that will die of terminal ridiculousness in three months. Bonus: You get to say "how vulgar" a lot, which can be fun, and the payoff—the aforementioned elegance—is huge.

**Look for pure shapes:** In the hope of camouflaging figure "flaws" (whether real or not), women often buy clothes whose basic shapes are obscured by ruffles, draping, layering, and general sagginess. If you want to build a classic wardrobe, resist this instinct to bury yourself, says celebrity stylist Jill Swid, who works with Uma Thurman. Trendy flourishes can actually make you look heavier, she says, and mark you as a fashion victim: "I hate extra fabric. I hate ruching. I always say, cleaner is better." Look for tailored shapes—a sheath dress, a pencil skirt—that give your body a clean silhouette. "On the red carpet," designer Olivier Theyskens has said of Nicole Kidman, "it is always Nicole, no matter who made the dress."

Okay, we know. That's fine for Nicole, whose body is a Platonic ideal, but what about the rest of you? The truth is clean tailoring makes most bodies look better. (Think how a Hugo Boss suit can turn a paunchy guy into a suave guy.) A classic sheath dress (a.k.a a fitted shift) works on most figures that are relatively proportionate top and bottom, whether straight or curvy. And a well-cut suit, with a nipped-in waist and a jacket that ends no lower than mid-hip, can make any woman look chic.

## Q.

### HOW CAN I LOOSEN UP THE CLASSICS?

Go ahead and break the rules, says Uma Thurman's stylist, **Jill Swid**, just keep it subtle. Some of her favorite twists:

❊ **Jolt a somber suit with colored driving gloves:** "Lavender, bright red, apple green…baby blue is beautiful if you're wearing brown."

❊ **Flash a lacy bra:** "With a classic white shirt, you want a little peekaboo. A little lace going on…a classic ladylike bra in a neutral. I'm not talking Frederick's of Hollywood."

❊ **Mix in denim:** "I love to wear this really old, soft, faded Wrangler denim shirt under my black Alexander McQueen tux. It's not too heavy, and the pearlized snap buttons are beautiful."

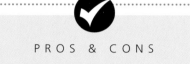

### PROS & CONS

#### CLASSIC LASTS

❊ **It's reliably chic:** This style has an eternal elegance that's hard to mess up. If you play (mostly) by the rules, you'll always look like a polished *somebody*.

❊ **In the long run, it's affordable:** Classic investment pieces are cost-efficient. Unlike a knockoff Chloë top, a $200 cashmere turtleneck works forever.

❊ **It's flexible:** Since classic pieces are simple, they function as wardrobe building blocks, easy to shake up with trendier accessories, to dress up, or dress down.

#### BUT WATCH OUT...

❊ **It's not the sexiest look:** Worn wrong, it can look uptight and overly formal. Look for skirts with slits, and unbutton that shirt (within reason) after dark.

❊ **It can make you look old before your time:** Avoid blouses with bows, heavier fabrics, Sasquatchy tweeds, boxy suits, and anything overly severe.

❊ **It's not the most expressive style:** If you really love inventing your own look, look elsewhere. But that doesn't mean you can't go classic once in a while—or wear it your own way.

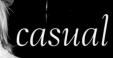

*casual*

**BRITNEY SPEARS**
With jeans and aviator shades, a turtleneck can make even Britney look sharp. Instant sophistication colors: black, white, or taupe.

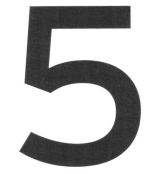

# 5
## ways to wear a turtleneck

Originally a thick, brutish sweater for thick, brutish men, it has become a feminine classic —and one of the planet's most versatile pieces.

**GWYNETH PALTROW**
A timeless formula: Start with a tweed pencil skirt (this one is Valentino), add a cashmere t-neck, and lean "I mean business" boots.

*urban chic*

*sexy*

**CHARLIZE THERON**
She'd look good in seaweed, but if you've got the legs, a t-neck over a fluttery mini—like this Alexander McQueen skirt—equals heat.

**UMA THURMAN**
Wow, right? Could this look be any prettier? Uma skims a powder-blue wool turtleneck over a pleated chiffon skirt by Luisa Beccaria.

*romantic*

**NAOMI WATTS**
A matchy look like this can seem uptight, but Naomi twists it with a bulky, almost outdoorsy, sweater.

*polished*

And don't forget color. A simple gown that might expose lumpiness in orange or baby blue can look lean in (you guessed it) black. **Other key shapes:** A-line dresses and skirts, straight-legged trousers, simple white shirts that aren't too blousy (Swid's favorite is by Thomas Pink). **Not classic:** Shape-handicapped clothes with no waist (trapeze dresses, for instance), stovepipe jeans, cargo-style anything.

**Make sure your clothes fit:** Don't buy a size too small, hoping to eventually carb-deny your way into it. Or a size too big, assuming it will be "forgiving." And don't obsess about size numbers; they're never consistent from store to store. Part of the reason stars look freakishly good more often than not: Their clothes fit. They skim the body, neither too tight nor too loose. The seams lie flat, the necklines don't gape, the garments' shoulders hug the stars' shoulders.

"Everything is about fit," says Swid. "I've found that women feel better and sexier when they're in clothing that embraces the body." She says it was tough convincing Uma to try skirt suits. The *Kill Bill* star dismissed the idea as dowdy, even when Swid showed her two strategically foxy tailored suits, a Valentino and a Chanel. "Uma's style is very ladylike and elegant, and there's a flirtatious feel to it. I'd never want it to look boxy," Swid says. "But she still said, 'No way, I am not wearing a skirt suit.' I said, 'Trust me.' And, listen, when she finally put them on? She turned to me and said, "How could a skirt suit work like this?"

Good fit is not reserved for those who can swing Chanel, according to Mary Alice Stephenson, Liv Tyler's stylist and the former fashion director of *Harper's Bazaar*: "It's true that women bought too big for years, but the clothes weren't tailored very well," she says. "Clothes, in general, are better cut now, so there's really no excuse."

## Suit Style 101

# STAID VS. SEXY

Depending on the cut, a skirt suit can make you look like a librarian...or a va-va-voomarian.

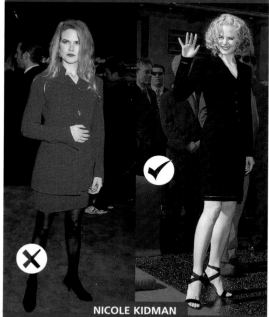

**NICOLE KIDMAN**

**STAID:** Nicole gets it *Working Girl*–wrong in an '80s-style jacket that's too long, bulking up her hips.

**SEXY:** A perfect length, this streamlined jacket looks even leaner in black with skyscraper heels.

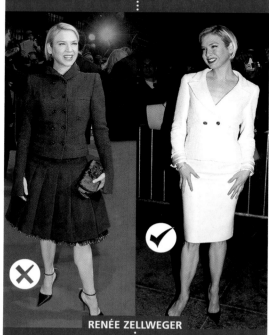

**RENÉE ZELLWEGER**

**STAID:** Despite a flirty tulle underlay, this stiff A-line suit looks like armor, overpowering Renee's graceful shoes.

**SEXY:** The frump factor is gone, thanks to a supple fitted suit with a pencil skirt and open neckline.

**Stick to a simple palette of solid colors:** The key trio is black, white, and camel. But unless you're brutally self-denying, you'll include cream, gray, navy blue, pink, and other ladylike pastels. And for those less ladylike moments, red. **Less classic:** Green, orange, yellow, turquoise. These are great for casual preppie looks—a linen summer shift or capri pants—or as a bold handbag accent, but generally too Crayola for dinner or cocktails. **Just no:** Most metallics (except for accessories), purple, neons.

**Use prints discriminatingly:** Jacqueline Kennedy wrote to a trusted fashion advisor in 1960, "Just remember that I like...terribly simple clothes," adding, "And I hate prints." Loudness isn't classic, so if you love prints, keep them quiet. The focus should be the garment's shape, and you. **Most classic:** Pretty florals, simple stripes or pinstripes, preppy plaids, tweed, herringbone, houndstooth, smaller polka dots. **Least classic:** Graphic geometry, trippy swirls, anything seemingly fingerpainted by an especially klutzy 5-year-old, except maybe as a scarf. A well-hidden scarf.

**Choose restrained accessories:** While you're busy elegantly refusing flashiness, remember to choose shoes, bags, and jewelry that will strengthen the total power effect, not beg for attention. "The reason Nicole Kidman looks so good," says Stephenson, "is that it all adds up to one 'wow' moment. It's not 'who made that belt, what's that bag?' It's the overall effect. When you see someone who didn't get it right, you see the elements, not the whole."

## LABELS TO LOOK FOR

**Designer:** Chanel, Carolina Herrera, Narciso Rodriguez, Michael Kors, Vera Wang.
**More Affordable:** Ann Taylor, Banana Republic, Anne Klein, Ellen Tracy, The Limited.

## Sweet Updo

"Because it was a sculptural dress," says celebrity hairstylist Kevin Mancuso, "I set it off with a sculptural, asymmetric updo, very Grace Kelly. I pulled her hair back into pigtails, then twisted them into two little buns like seashells."

## Aristocratic Rocks

Renée wore $1 million worth of Cartier jewels, including a 73-carat oval-and-pear-shaped diamond necklace with a 35-carat diamond bracelet.

## '30s Couture Draping

Inspired by antiquity, French couturiers such as Madame Gres (whose dream to be a sculptor was squashed by her loser parents) began designing by draping and pinning silk directly on a woman's body. Her influence is obvious in Renée's "wrapped" satin bodice.

# ANATOMY OF
# A GOWN

*Renée Zellweger* in Carolina Herrera at the 2004 Oscars: *Classic glamour—part '30s Parisian couture, part Marilyn Monroe—wrapped up with a gorgeous goliath of a train.*

## Gentlemen Prefer Giant Bows

"My dress felt like old Hollywood glamour," Renée commented. One likely reference point: The pink gown Marilyn Monroe wears while befriending diamonds in *Gentlemen Prefer Blondes* (1953). In both cases, a restrained column shape erupts into an extravagant bow.

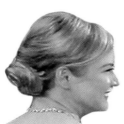

## The Train

Designer Carolina Herrera ingeniously extended the bow's "ends" into a two-tiered, four-foot train for full-throttle glamour. "I felt nervous for my train," Renée has said, and later admitted she still feels awed by such masterpiece gowns: "I [think], Oh, my God. I know what went into that, and that's not five minutes at the sewing machine. It's a lot of dreaming and planning."

## Body-Conscious Fit

Renée was 25 pounds overweight after portraying Bridget Jones, but Carolina Herrera advised her to play up her curves rather than shrouding her body in a shapeless gown.

# The Elements of Style

Polish the look with well-bred accessories: a pump with Nicole pedigree, Renée-worthy gloves, and (blow that inheritance!) the holy grail, an Hermès bag.

THE BIRKIN BAG It's not the most classic of the hand-crafted Hermès bags—that would be the smaller, boxier Kelly Bag, which Grace Kelly wielded to shield her pregnancy from nosy paparazzi in 1956. For Catherine Zeta-Jones, Lucy Lui, and other understated stars, however, the slouchier and surprisingly roomy Birkin (b. 1984) is the must-Hermès. Craftsmen train for five years before they're allowed to handstitch a Birkin (an 18-hour process) out of classic cowhide, immodest sharkskin, even goat. Does this justify the cost (up to $20,000) or a waiting list that has left Birkin hopefuls languishing for two years? Well, no. But patience is a classic virtue.

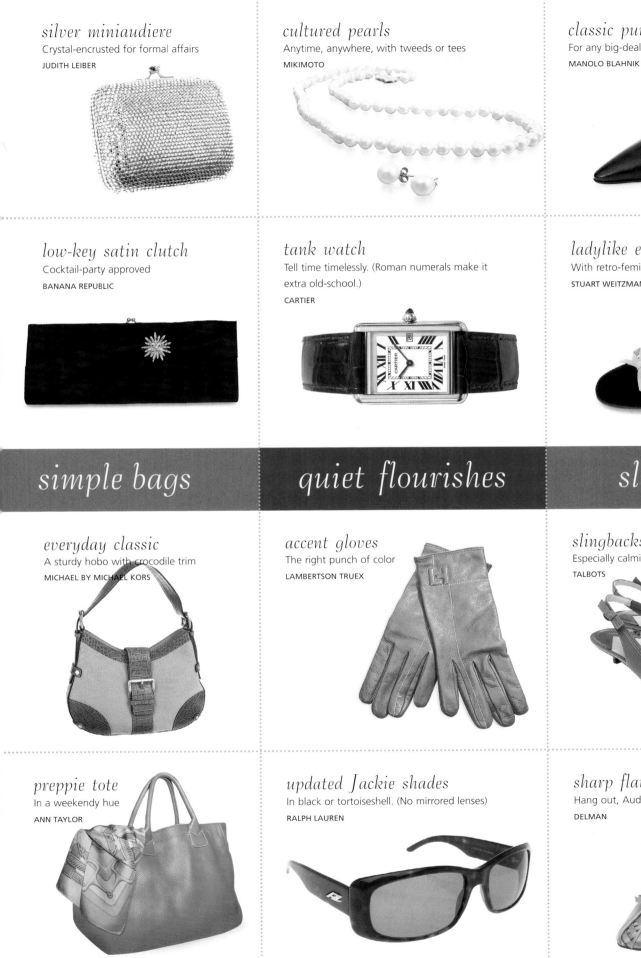

### silver miniaudiere
Crystal-encrusted for formal affairs
JUDITH LEIBER

### cultured pearls
Anytime, anywhere, with tweeds or tees
MIKIMOTO

### classic pumps
For any big-deal occasion
MANOLO BLAHNIK

### low-key satin clutch
Cocktail-party approved
BANANA REPUBLIC

### tank watch
Tell time timelessly. (Roman numerals make it extra old-school.)
CARTIER

### ladylike evening shoes
With retro-feminine details
STUART WEITZMAN

## simple bags

## quiet flourishes

## sleek shoes

### everyday classic
A sturdy hobo with crocodile trim
MICHAEL BY MICHAEL KORS

### accent gloves
The right punch of color
LAMBERTSON TRUEX

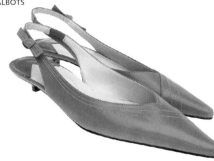

### slingbacks
Especially calming in camel for stressful days
TALBOTS

### preppie tote
In a weekendy hue
ANN TAYLOR

### updated Jackie shades
In black or tortoiseshell. (No mirrored lenses)
RALPH LAUREN

### sharp flats
Hang out, Audrey-style, in pure prettiness.
DELMAN

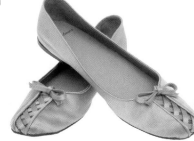

# chapter 3

# CREATIVE

True creative chic is about mixing it up—and it's never a snore. In the No-Doz style of **Kirsten Dunst** and **Sarah Jessica Parker**, seemingly incompatible ideas find happiness together. Burnt-orange hangs out with pink. Tweed itches for satin. Seventies wedgies give '30s gowns an unexpected boost. Creative dressers don't just tug clothes off hangers, they play with possibilities. (Suspenders for evening: Check!) This look has no standard rulebook. It takes a scenic detour—with stops at vintage stores and guys' closets—past the "good taste" comfort zone of cream, camel, and black. If it's your style, you've never had much use for rules anyway. (Except maybe that "no nylons with sandals" thing.) Inspiration, on the other hand? Always cool with that.

"I'm the kind of girl who wears flip-flops to the Chateau Marmont."

—KIRSTEN DUNST

# Sarah Jessica Parker

Once besotted with trends, Sarah has learned to wear fashion her way—
**cooly chaotic**, mixed with vintage, and never straight off the runway.

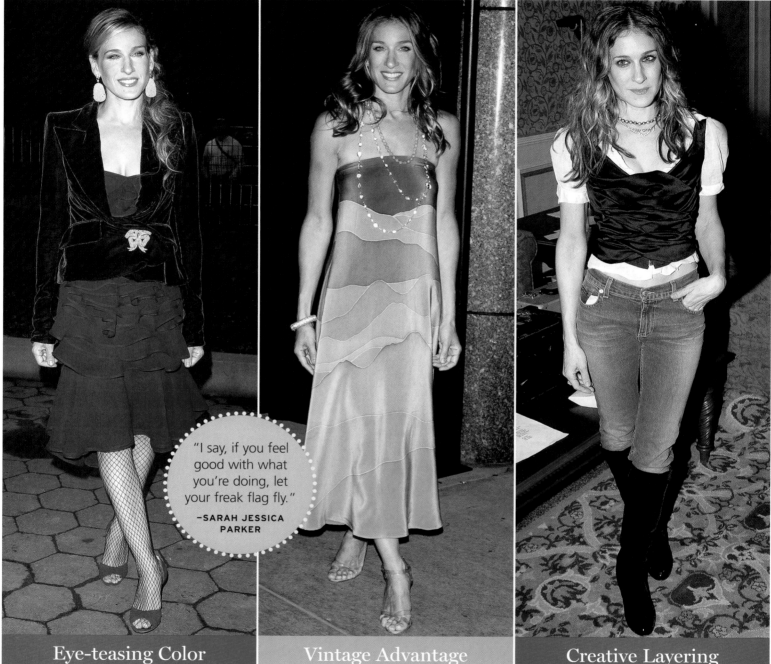

> "I say, if you feel good with what you're doing, let your freak flag fly."
> —SARAH JESSICA PARKER

## Eye-teasing Color

## Vintage Advantage

## Creative Layering

A more cautious woman would have worn this YSL Rive Gauche outfit with neutral accessories, but Sarah Jessica zings it with hits of turquoise and red peep-toe shoes.

For antigeneric chic, work vintage pieces into your wardrobe. SJP loves the '50s formal look, but tries on another era in this '70s batik skimmer—looped with a dynamic necklace duo.

Sarah Jessica glams up an innocent muslin top by adding a second one in sexy black satin. Love it or hate it, you have to admire her indifference to what we think.

# Cate Blanchett

Sophisticated. Theatrical. Complex. Bohemian.
No one word can sum up Cate's **eclectic style**—and she likes it that way.

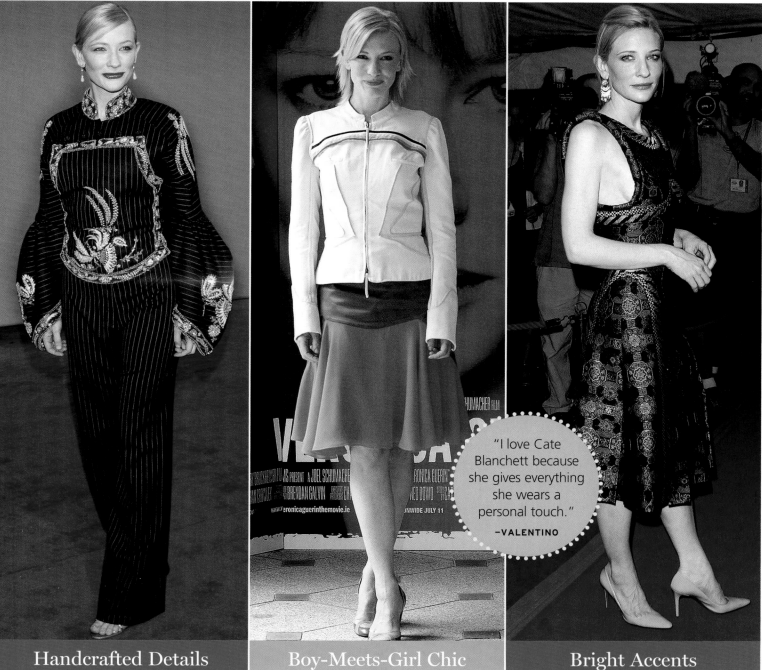

> "I love Cate Blanchett because she gives everything she wears a personal touch."
> —VALENTINO

## Handcrafted Details

Creatives like crafty adornment, especially if it's used in unfolksy ways. Case in point: Cate's pin-striped Christian Dior Couture pantsuit with Chinoiserie embroidery.

## Boy-Meets-Girl Chic

Contrasting two opposite ideas (formal/casual or masculine/feminine) is key to creative style. A modified motorcycle jacket, complete with racing stripes, toughs up Cate's fluttery dress.

## Bright Accents

It's just as kickass to hit one color note strongly as to play with several shades. An easy trick: wake up an overly "respectable" gray dress with Miami-blue stilettos.

# Kirsten Dunst

Winsome, sexy, and instinctively stylish, Kirsten makes taking risks seem easy and—despite the **rare "huh?" outfit**—so very worth it.

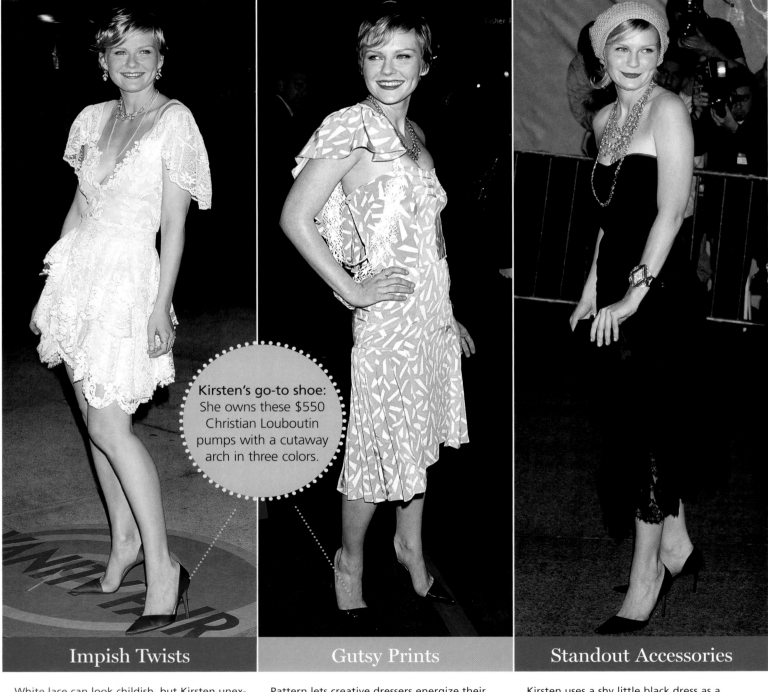

Kirsten's go-to shoe: She owns these $550 Christian Louboutin pumps with a cutaway arch in three colors.

## Impish Twists

## Gutsy Prints

## Standout Accessories

White lace can look childish, but Kirsten unexpectedly sexes it up with this Christian Lacroix minidress. (Petal sleeves and 19th-century gems keep it anti-Britney.)

Pattern lets creative dressers energize their look. On this retro dress, designed by Milla Jovovich, snips of white skip across aqua—playful yet sharp, like Kirsten herself.

Kirsten uses a shy little black dress as a canvas to showcase a bravura Deco bracelet, five strands of gems, and (nervy!) a crocheted beret, more typically a day look.

# [Street Glam Slam!]

*Street glam is the bratty little sister to creative style: Louder, more audacious, and heavy on the attitude. The mix is different—retro sweetness out, urban fierceness in.*

### Ashanti ➤
**in BONDAGE CHIC**

Not that any of that hardware on her pants is functional, but don't you get the impression that Ashanti could fix plumbing in this and still look hot?

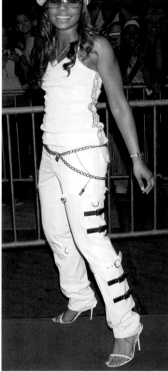

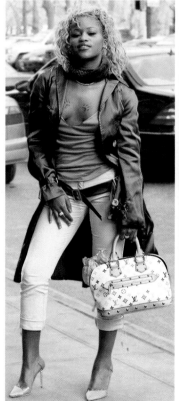

### ◄ Eve
**working LOUIS VUITTON**

There's a lot going on here—satin, plastic, a fashion-victimy Vuitton Murakami bag. But it works, thanks to Eve's color-mixing confidence and her swagger.

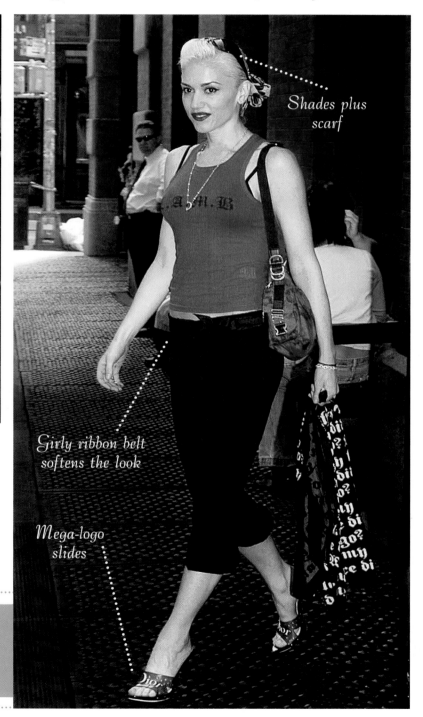

*Shades plus scarf*

*Girly ribbon belt softens the look*

*Mega-logo slides*

### Gwen Stefani in CHRISTIAN DIOR ➤

The rock fashionista gives a red tank and Dior mules her trademark "je ne sais *yeah*" styling. One part Rizzo from *Grease*. One part shopaholic. Two parts "Take my picture, sucker."

# MADONNA

## Patron Saint of Style

# Rowdy Layering

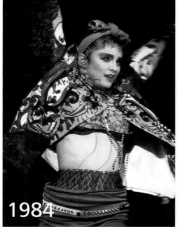

1984

MADONNA

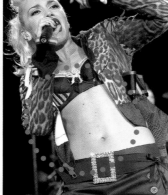

2004

GWEN STEFANI

············· Eighties Excess ·············

**Then:** In her early days, Madonna's style was clearly "More is more!" She mixed "innocent" bows and vampy lingerie with a Reagan-era wink. **Now:** Gwen Stefani's updated blend, just as manic but less coy.

············· Skank to Goddess ·············

**Then:** Continually rebranding herself, Madonna has created over 12 images, including Skunk-haired Hussy (top) and Blonde Bombshell (below). Her '80s "Material Girl" homage to Marilyn Monroe (revisited in 1998) helped trigger Hollywood's full-scale return to classic glamour. **Now:** Makeover junkie Christina Aguilera lamely Xeroxes the same looks.

## Strategic Makeovers

**m**odern creative chic certainly didn't start with Madonna. In the '40s, bohemians paired perfectly cut French suits with chunky peasant jewelry. Twenty years later, hippies invented their own vintage mix of old and nude. And, circa 1976, London punks safety-pinned themselves into fashion history. But it was the big M who shoved the idea of "styling yourself" so far into the mainstream that it stuck. (Macy's once transformed an entire sales floor into "Madonnaland.") Born in Michigan, she grew up in a prison of plainness—her stepmother made her wear the same dull dresses as her sisters—but she instinctively rebelled, flashing fuchsia panties under her school-uniform skirt and performing nearly naked at talent shows. Eventually she fled to New York City where she scavenged through thrift stores to create her early-'80s Boy Toy look. Ripped shirts. Men's trousers. Minis over fishnet bodysuits. Rags to rooster-ify her hair, which she slathered in olive oil to keep matted. On her dancer's body, this mix worked. On the scrawny teenyboppers who soon emulated her? Not so much. But the point—that pretty much anything goes—helped transform style irreversibly.

As a true creative, Madonna quickly moved on, constantly reinventing her look to remain unique. Ask yourself: How many celebrities have been married in a white veil topped by a black bowler hat? Answer: One.

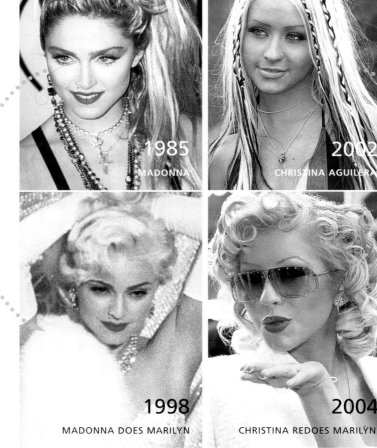

1985
MADONNA

2002
CHRISTINA AGUILERA

1998
MADONNA DOES MARILYN

2004
CHRISTINA REDOES MARILYN

# get the look

If your wardrobe has become too numblingly routine, start thinking like Hollywood's style innovators. "Boring" is the only look they just can't risk.

**For some women, getting dressed is just routine problem-solving.** Black clothes for work, jeans for a bar, a T-shirt to bed. Whenever one of their friends gets married, they drag out the regulation slip-dress with 2.2 rosebuds per square inch. Creative dressers are quite the opposite; unless they're crazy-busy, they always welcome a chance to invent an outfit. If you're not feeling confident about your ability to throw random pieces together with Kirstenesque verve, we're here to say, "Get over it." Sure there are no rules to guarantee you'll get it right, but what are you, a woman or a generically dressed mouse?

**Start experimenting:** "Creative style is about play and taking risks," says stylist Mary Alice Stephenson, the former fashion director of *Harper's Bazaar*, who works with the notably risk-taking Liv Tyler. "If you look at Kirsten Dunst, you never think...oh, she's wearing Marc Jacobs or Valentino. You just think she had all those things in her closet, and she had a lot of fun putting them together."

Merely replicating some "creative" designer's runway look from head to toe is too obvious. "I don't put people in one of those trademark Pucci dresses or in Missoni because it's so detectable," says celebrity stylist Jill Swid. "It's always so 'oh my god, that's Missoni.'" The goal is to find your own mix. So give yourself time to play.

Turn off that compelling Lifetime movie about twin psychic dog-breeders, and devote an hour to trying new style combos. Banish all

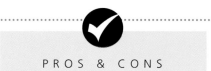

## PROS & CONS

### YAY, CREATIVE!

✳ **Creative style is memorable:** People who make strong impressions get wonderful things like parts in movies and free rides home from parties.

✳ **It can be very affordable:** Especially if you work the thrift stores, steal from men's closets, and take your mom's old college dresses to the tailor.

✳ **It's the most modern way to dress:** Creative is the insider's style—flexible, as multifaceted as pop culture. If you do it well, you won't look obviously "in" or "out" of fashion.

### BUT WATCH OUT...

✳ **It's easy to go overboard:** What happens when that daring pattern mix suddenly looks dubious at the party? Well, sometimes dubious beats boring. Otherwise, surreptitiously dim the lights.

✳ **Excessive layering can look frumpy:** A scarf over a capelet over a military jacket over a sweater can be a very bad thing. Keep it sexy: Remember skin?

✳ **It's harder to pull off for work:** Unless you work in one of the less stodgy fields, the old backward-sweater trick may be more trouble than it's worth.

men, kids, and know-it-all friends. If you think a top is supposed to be worn alone over skin, slip it over a long-sleeved fitted tee. Casualize a velvet skirt with a T-shirt. Do something deliberately "incorrect." (Wear a loose, drapey sweater backwards. Try boots with a summer dress or khaki shorts, even a nightgown.) If you find a mix you like, wear it out next weekend. Promise?

"Sometimes you do get it wrong," says Stephenson. "Look back at Sarah Jessica in the '80s. Wow, did she get it wrong. But every time, you'll learn from it and find your way. If there's anything I've learned working with celebrities, it's that you can't please everyone. No one is scrutinized as brutally as they are . . . and you'll never satisfy all the critics."

**Show trends who's boss:** Creative dressers sniff out each new trend for the stench of "fashion victim." If you truly like a look, mix it in with your beloved older pieces. But if you find this year's "it" bags indefensibly fugly, go with something plainer, and style around it. Maybe your twist comes from a cute vintage skirt, or an idiosyncratic top by a local designer. And don't overspend on trends; with the exception of shoes, that cheaper version will last as long as you need it.

Remember: Most must-have fads are like dandelions. They may root themselves in fashion with weedlike power, but when the season's over, they blow away. When Sarah Jessica Parker succumbed to the Louis Vuitton Murakami bag, a hot item in 2003,

**ALICIA KEYS**

✓ The dress-over-jeans look is a love/hate thing, but this pattern mix is definitely working (It's easier to mix patterns of similar color.)

✗ Wearing jeans *over* a dress, on the other hand? This experiment looks more like open-gown surgery than fashion.

**MAGGIE GYLLENHAAL**

✓ Maggie adapts the exaggerated proportions of the '80s—tiny puffed skirt, wide shoulders—without looking misshapen.

✗ A flight suit plus Ugg boots equals Trend Victim 2003. (Is her left hand is too ashamed to be seen with her?)

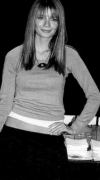

# 5
## stars who went too far

✓ *creative*    ✗ *too creative*

When the mix is beginning to look schlubby, gaudy, or escaped-mental-patient-y, it's time to put down the hanger.

**MISCHA BARTON**

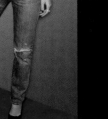

✓ With the simple addition of a little gold jacket, Mischa turns a routine jeans look into nightclub-ready modern glam.

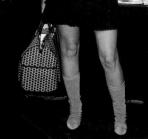

✗ Mischa pays a high price for warm ankles in a layered, legging look that chops her body into too many pieces.

**KIRSTEN DUNST**

✓ Texture play: A heavy, nubbly cardigan looks great slung over a flouncy dress. Buttoning it "wrong" only makes it sexier.

✗ Kirsten has often mixed black leggings into dressed-down looks, usually with cuter results than this.

**EVE**

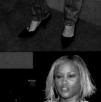

✓ You might think pink paisley and an Asian floral print would quarrel, but Eve calms the combo with soothing cream capris.

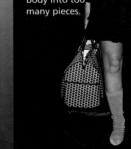

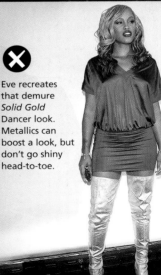

✗ Eve recreates that demure *Solid Gold* Dancer look. Metallics can boost a look, but don't go shiny head-to-toe.

she knew its Japanese adorability would soon fade. "I'm not going to be precious with this bag," she declared at the time. "Pat Field [her *Sex and the City* stylist] told me to burn it, to run it into the ground. I mean, can you wear it after this season?" In a word: no.

**Let vintage be your friend:** Unique looks start with one-of-a-kind pieces, so think beyond the mall. Try the retro shopping options: garage sales, thrift stores, premium vintage stores like New York Vintage in Manhattan, or Los Angeles's Decades. Natalie Portman likes to tweak her classic style with vintage scores like a '60s V-neck sweater depicting an owl: "On one arm it says 'Some are wise,' " she's said, "and on the other arm, it says 'Some are otherwise.' " Vintage finds let you be both.

**Use accessories to "flip" a look:** If you play against type, bags or jewelry can change an outfit's personality. With a preppy twin-set, try funky hoop earrings instead of pearls. (Save the pearls to wear with a protest tee.)

---

ENTRY-LEVEL STYLE

## SIX SIMPLE WAYS TO MIX IT UP

Reblend your look with these eclectic styling tricks, all star-tested.

✳ Throw on a jean jacket over a floral dress. Very **Uma Thurman**.

✳ Wear silver round-toe shoes with jeans during the day à la **Mischa Barton**.

✳ Carry a vintage embroidered bag to breakfast in **Cate Blanchett** fashion.

✳ De-Gap a tee with real jewelry. **Drew Barrymore** gets into coral.

✳ Sling a jeans-y leather belt over a fluttery dress, a **Kirsten Dunst** move.

✳ Wear two contrasting necklaces (say, wooden and crystal beads) like **SJP**.

---

**Mix textures:** When it comes to various kinds of mixing, here's the degree of difficulty: 1) **Graphic prints:** Really tough. Good luck with that. 2) **Subtler prints:** Risky, but cool in a Milla Jovovich way (think pinstripes with a vintage floral). 3) **Color:** Easy if a neutral shade is involved (orange plus gray). Trickier when you're combining two vivid colors. 4) **Texture:** The easiest mix. Textures equal in weight (corduroy and velvet) go together naturally, but it's more surprising and sensual to switch it up. Corduroy and silk? Velvet and chiffon? And then there's the Pandora's box of sequins, fur, mock-crocodile...

Don't overdo it, cautions Stephenson. "It's great to mix two different textures, say, a cotton ribbed tank and a little sequined jacket. But you don't also need to wear some amazing textural patchwork socks."

### LABELS TO LOOK FOR

**Designer:** Marc Jacobs, Christian Dior, Miu-Miu, Chloe, Stella McCartney, Proenza Schouler
**More Affordable:** H&M, Bebe, Anthropologie, Urban Outfitters, thrift and vintage options

---

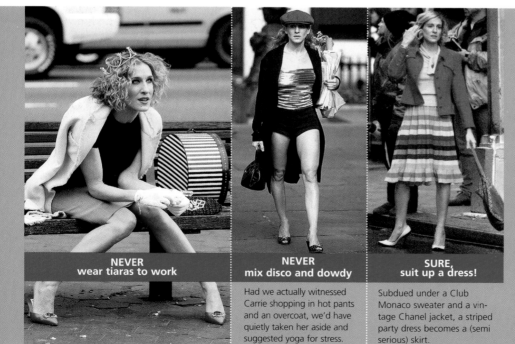

**NEVER**
wear tiaras to work

**NEVER**
mix disco and dowdy

Had we actually witnessed Carrie shopping in hot pants and an overcoat, we'd have quietly taken her aside and suggested yoga for stress.

**SURE,**
suit up a dress!

Subdued under a Club Monaco sweater and a vintage Chanel jacket, a striped party dress becomes a (semi serious) skirt.

## SEX AND THE ECCENTRICITY

Creative style lessons from *Sex and the City*—the most relentlessly chic show in television history.

As *SATC*'s style pioneer Carrie Bradshaw from 1998 to 2004, Sarah Jessica Parker sometimes changed outfits more than 10 times an episode, recklessly triggering trends (giant, sneeze-inducing silk flower, anyone?). Her head-held-high willingness to wear *anything*—remember the tutu?—encouraged ordinary women to take their own fashion risks. The mix, concocted by the show's costume designer Patricia Field, changed Sarah Jessica's personal style, too. Without it, she's said, "I think [my look] would have been more conservative, and I'm far more conservative than the character."

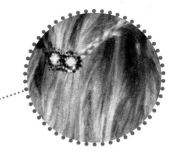

### "Undone" Hair

Critics carped at Cate's "messy" hair-style, missing the point: With its mini-braids and deliberately uneven part, it has a fresh maiden vibe in tune with her gown. The clips? "They're actually earrings," says Pastor, "but we ended up sewing them into her hair."

### Dreaming Up the Dress

Soon after she was nominated for *Elizabeth*, Cate and her stylist, Jessica Pastor, sat with designer John Galliano at a London restaurant, poring over "look books" of his past collections, picking ingredients they hoped to combine: "It could be a stitching, a neckline," says Pastor, who's worked with Cate since 1997. "She's always had a very cool, eclectic chic."

# ANATOMY OF
# A GOWN

*Cate Blanchett in John Galliano for Dior at the 1999 Oscars: Embroidered blossoms. Enamored birds. Years ahead of its time, this fairy tale of a dress redefined "unique."*

### Smear Tactics

"I originally wanted the flowers air-brushed in paint," says Pastor, who admits it was a "very bad" idea. "But we realized it would smear when people hugged her. That's when the embroidery came in." It took two months to complete.

### The Ideal Gems

Pastor traveled "all over the world" looking for jewelry that wouldn't overwhelm the dress's whimsy, before she found these amethyst flower bracelets from legendary British jewelers Asprey & Garrard's Daisy collection.

### Hummingbirds in Love

"We asked John to create a love story with this dress. Not everyone noticed this, but there's a second hummingbird," Pastor points out, lurking in the fishtail hem. "I've always thought they were chirping to each other."

# Uncommon Touches

Give any look a tender twist with an unexpected clutch, a cloche hat, or that cornerstone of Sarah Jessica chic: the collectible shoe.

RISING STARS These Miu Miu satin Mary Janes have the sort of energetic retro charm that attracts a true shoe fetishist like Sarah Jessica Parker, who's admitted she owns roughly 60 pairs: "That's if you're talking about the shoes in circulation, because I have an archive, too." Collectible shoes are an investment a creative dresser knows she'll wear whenever they find their way into her mix, whether tomorrow, next fall, or in 10 years. Which isn't to say you have to spend a ton on every pair. But if you want versatile keepers, look for beauty, look for character, and not just fleeting cool.

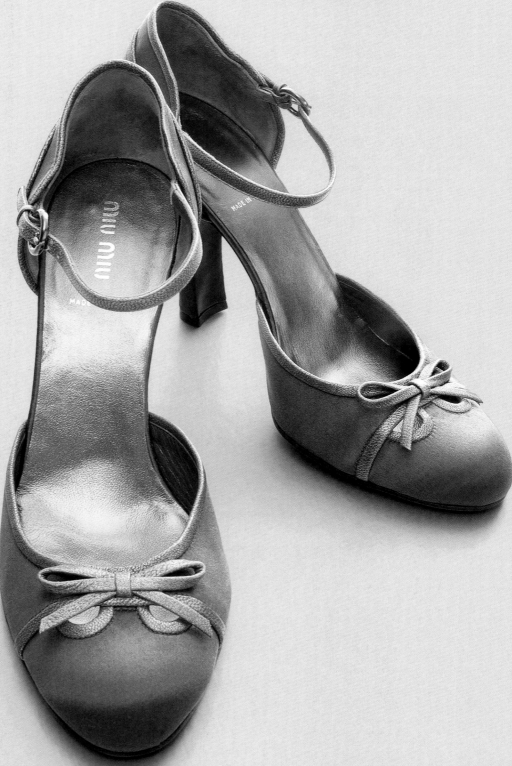

### embellished evening bag
Plain has its moments, but...not just now.

JAMIN PUECH

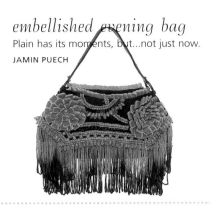

### nostalgic jewelry
From a retro broach to a vintage engagement ring

ALEX AND ANI

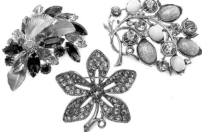

### anti-boring stilettos
Try Kelly green suede—dressy doesn't mean black.

BRIAN ATWOOD

### club-friendly clutch
Strawberries...straw bag...coincidence?

LULU GUINNESS

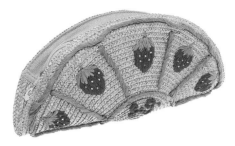

### cunning key chains
Express your personal style...inside your bag.

MOSCHINO

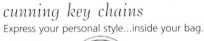

### crafty soles
Texture mixes add richness from the ground up.

MOSCHINO

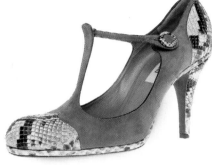

## playful bags

## eclectic extras

## statement shoes

### jolty satchel
Brighten even the most tedious work days.

MARC JACOBS

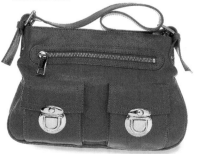

### mad hats
Most women fear them. You can pull them off.

MICHELLE DEBORAH

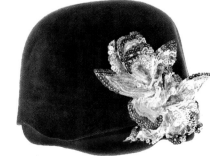

### bow details
Totally unnecessary, but we're talking shoes, not dishwashers.

POLLINI

### charismatic tote
Creative pack-rats hoard in style.

BOTKIER

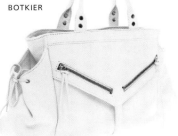

### futuristic shades
Why not? Too much retro gets predictable.

CHRISTIAN DIOR

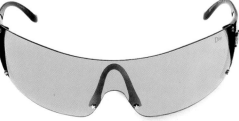

### unique sneaks
Old-school Adidas? Designer chic? You choose.

BANANA REPUBLIC

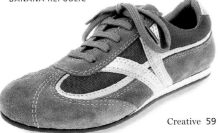

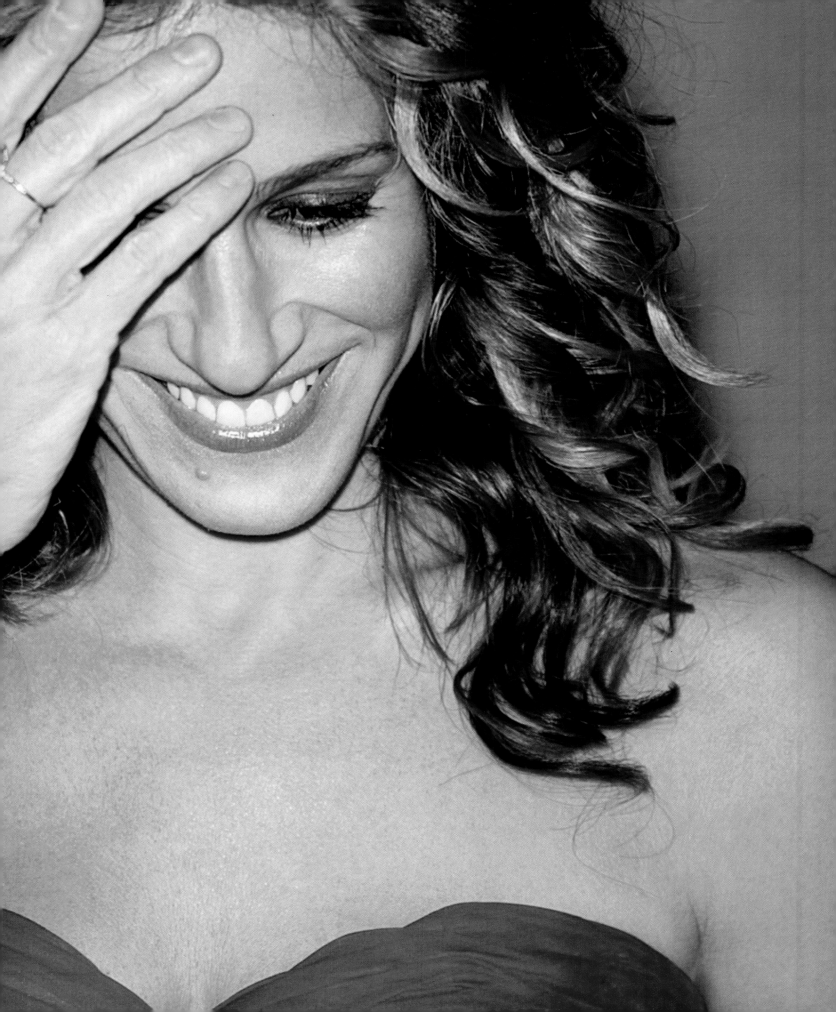

"I LEAVE NOTES SAYING, 'I APOLOGIZE FOR THE STATE OF THE CLOSET. I'LL CLEAN IT UP!'"

—SARAH JESSICA PARKER
ON THE MAYHEM SHE CREATES TRYING ON OUTFITS AT HOME

# chapter 4

# ALL-AMERICAN SEXY

## What makes style all-American?

Well, as obvious as it sounds…freedom. All-American sexy is the comfortable tomboy chic of **Jennifer Aniston** or **Cameron Diaz**. Sipping sake in a tank top. Red-carpet pants. Jersey dresses you can run in, fight in, scramble down a fire escape in—wear to bed. (All suitable for diving into pools.) What makes it sexy? The same things that make a woman wrapped in a plain white sheet sexy: Clothes so simple there's not much to distract from her natural accessories, her skin and hair. (Who needs a $1,100 bag?). Fabrics that move with you, that relent, that slip over shoulders if you do that shaking-with-laughter thing. For you, comfort is non-negotiable…even if it hasn't *always* looked amazing. Why not have both?

"Dude, I honestly don't know what
A-list means."

–CAMERON DIAZ

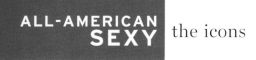

# Jennifer Aniston

Killer body. **No-fuss style.** Jennifer wears more black than a Supreme Court justice, but always finds a way to make it seriously sexy.

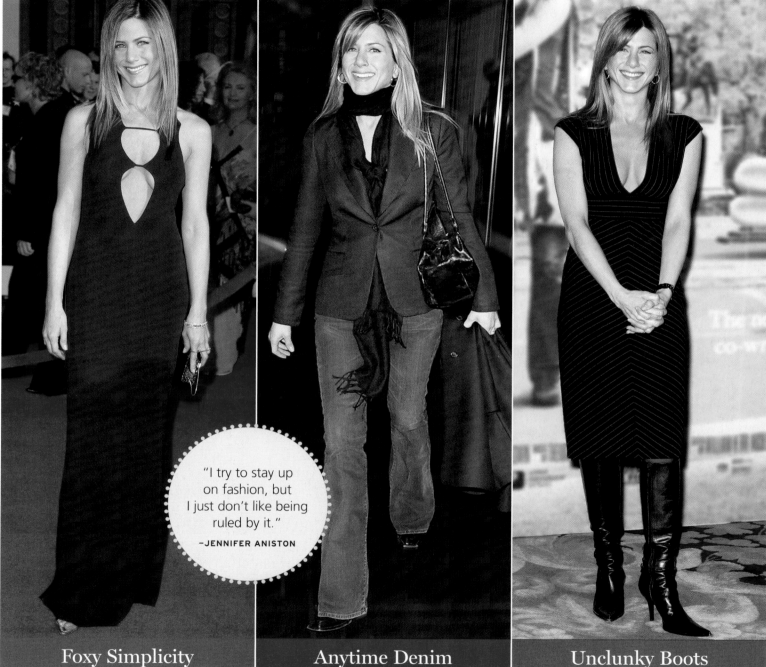

"I try to stay up on fashion, but I just don't like being ruled by it."

–JENNIFER ANISTON

**Foxy Simplicity**

**Anytime Denim**

**Unclunky Boots**

Jennifer on minimalism: "I love clothes where the body stands out." Rarely has hers stood out as sexily as in this Giorgio Armani gown with its cooperative cut-outs.

Why this dressy denim look works so well: Jen's jeans are as fitted as the jacket, dark (not overprocessed), and surrounded by a nuanced mix of lustrous black pieces.

Tall, elegant boots, the simpler the better, are key to all-American sexy style. Jennifer wears hers with a jersey dress in subtle pinstripes, which is about as patterned as she'll ever go.

# Cameron Diaz

Her style veers from hip eclecticism to sporty minimalism, but Cameron's spirit stays the same. The **sexy tomboy**: Surfer, winker, mover, shaker.

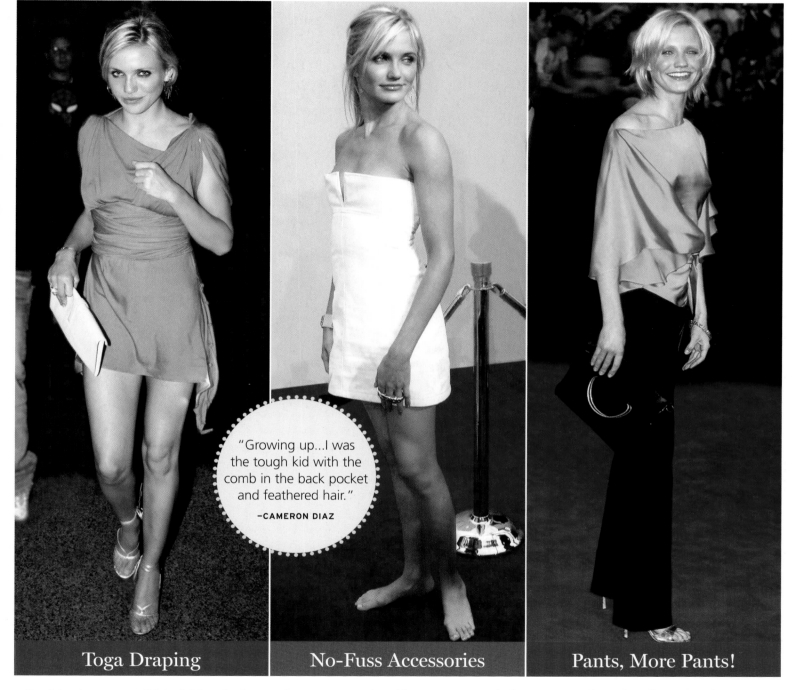

"Growing up...I was the tough kid with the comb in the back pocket and feathered hair."

—CAMERON DIAZ

## Toga Draping

## No-Fuss Accessories

## Pants, More Pants!

Greek huntresses weren't into tight, and neither are their American descendants. This easygoing minidress has been wrapped, knotted, and released back into the wild.

Cameron accessorizes this sweet gym-towel of a dress with hoop earings and little else. No brooches, necklaces, not even shoes. (Her sandals had just broken.)

Pants are the perfect all-American date or dinner party solution. Cameron distills the cute-top look into Amish simplicity in sleek trousers, topped by a silky wave of blue.

# Angelina Jolie

She lives in pants, but when Angelina needs a dress, she goes for one of the **modern American classics**—from the sweatshirt mini to the halter.

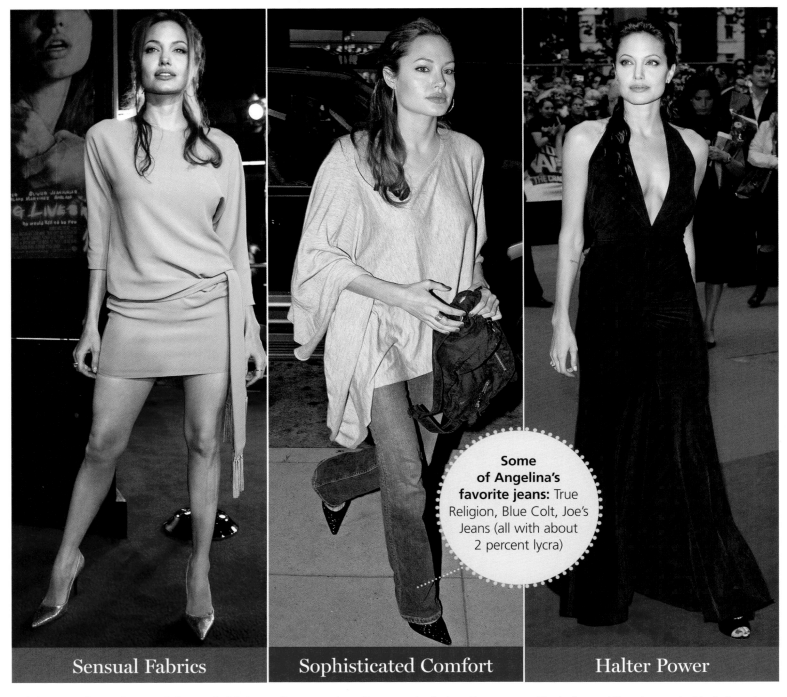

Some of Angelina's **favorite jeans:** True Religion, Blue Colt, Joe's Jeans (all with about 2 percent lycra)

### Sensual Fabrics

### Sophisticated Comfort

### Halter Power

A.A. sexy style gets its oomph from soft fabrics that drape amazingly but know just how to hug a thigh: silk, stretch wool, or jersey, like this neo-Flashdance minidress by Celine.

Texture and quality can make "relaxed" seem aristocratic. If Angelina's cashmere poncho were made of hemp, or her jeans cheaply "distressed", she wouldn't look this good.

The halter neckline plunges decisively, broadens shoulders, makes almost any woman look Amazonian—all very A.A. sexy. Its assertive glamour, in black silk, suits Angelina perfectly.

# [THE NIGHT-OUT SUIT]

*The essential all-American alternative to a dress:*
*White if you want to strut, black if you want to smolder,*
*and weird 'n' glitzy if you want to work for a circus.*

*Beach-blown hair*

*Strategic camisole*

*Body-conscious (but not suffocating) fit*

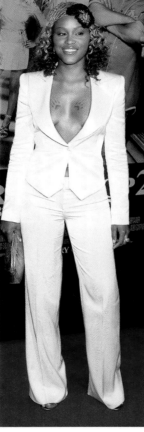

### ◄ Eve

In an edgy cut with a cleavage-hugging jacket, the white suit radiates an even fresher strength. Eve's crocheted cap pays homage to Ali McGraw's 1971 Oscars look.

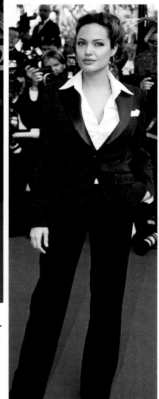

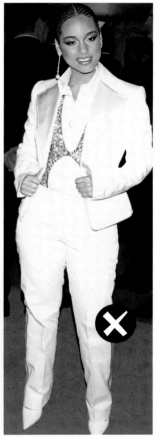

### Angelina Jolie ✈

In black, the tux has a sultrier vibe. Angelina powers up a Dolce & Gabbana version with a white men's-style shirt (note the wide-spread collar) and an unfussy updo.

### ✦ Alicia Keys

**ALL-AMERICAN UNSEXY:**
Even if you're a hip-hop star with bold nonconformist style, don't undermine a white suit with a cutaway glitter vest and matching white shoes.

### ◄ Naomi Watts

The modern white suit: simply accessorized, tailored so it isn't boxy, subtly sheeny, and revealing enough to blow off any whiff of "corporate."

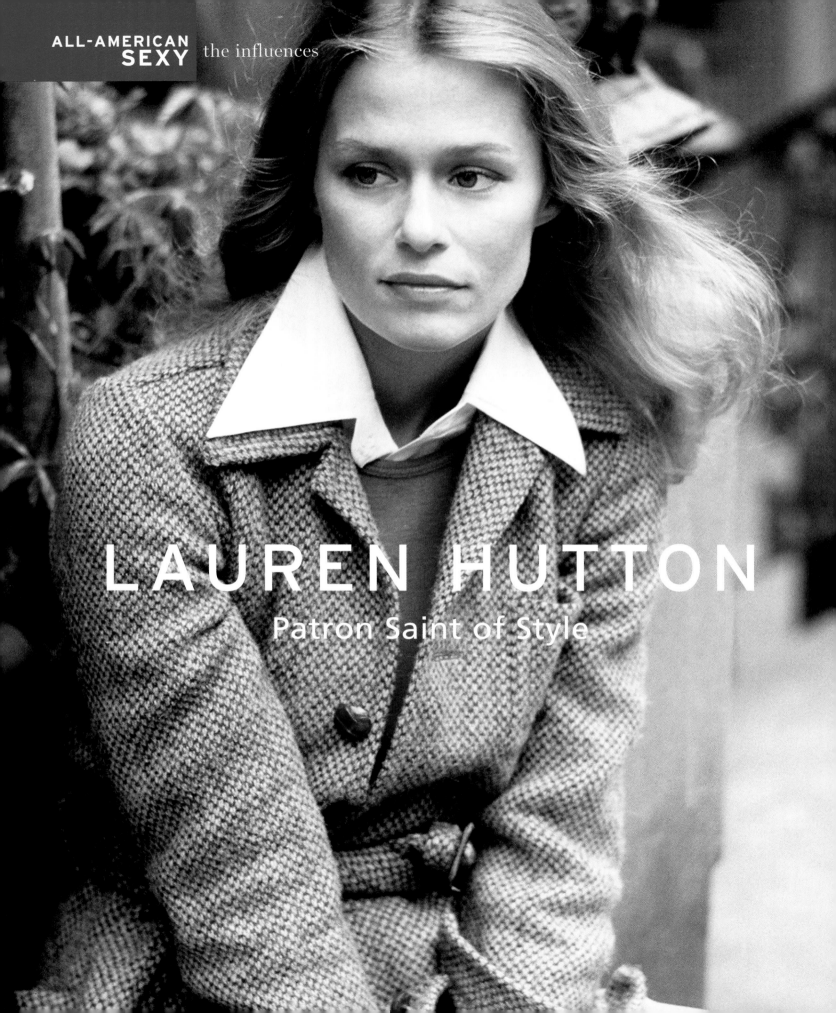

# LAUREN HUTTON

## Patron Saint of Style

**S**he was America's first supermodel, the one who famously refused to fix the gap in her teeth but bagged the big bucks anyway. Unpretentious and determined to be real, Lauren Hutton defined the natural early-'70s woman, and she stayed natural even as the rest of the nation overdosed on disco kitsch and '80s excess. She grew up in the Florida swamp, raising worms, slugging boys, happily beheading dolls—not the childhood of your typical style role model. Her mom, she's said, was a "major fashion freak" who dreamed of crocodile accessories and had her hair combed out every day. Lauren liked jeans. And T-shirts. Her biggest dream was to get to Kenya before all the zebra and rhinoceros were slaughtered.

## Sexy Suits

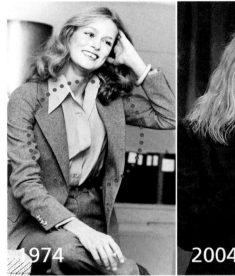

1974 — LAUREN HUTTON
2004 — DREW BARRYMORE

Fame was partly accidental. Stranded in mid-'60s New York, and scheming to survive until she could catch a tramp steamer to Africa, Lauren took a $50-a-week job as a serflike showroom model at Christian Dior. But fate intervened—in the form of *Vogue*'s legendary editor Diana Vreeland, who imperiously discovered her one afternoon during a routine fitting. (Lauren recalls one long finger pointed in her direction: "You!"). Soon she was booking major covers and, by 1973, had snagged an unprecedented million-dollar Ultima II cosmetics contract. Even at her peak, however, Lauren dressed as unfussily as possible off camera. Blazers. Jeans. More jeans. Slash-and-stun halter dresses. Plus: whatever she wore when she finally got to eat two-inch-long termites in the Congo. They taste, she's said, like "Brazil nuts."

## Bucket Caps

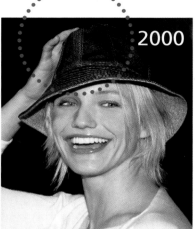

1980 — LAUREN HUTTON
2000 — CAMERON DIAZ

·············· **Laid-back Hats** ··············

**Then:** Lauren sports her signature faded canvas cap, and her gap-toothed grin. (Note blanket improvised as a cape.) **Now:** Equally toothy, Cameron Diaz updates the bucket in dark denim for night.

·············· **Suit Style** ··············

**Then:** For most women, the well-cut, nonsilly trouser suit wasn't an option until the '70s. Lauren showed them how to unbutton its serious side. **Now:** Fellow free spirit Drew Barrymore follows suit.

·············· **Plunging Necklines** ··············

**Then:** Influential '70s designer Halston draped women in clothes they could move in—perfect for Lauren, who wore his 1975 gown to the Oscars. **Now:** Maggie Gyllenhaal takes her own Halstonian plunge.

## Halter Gowns

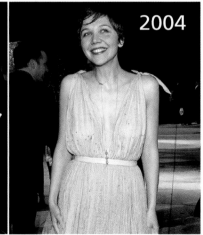

1975 — LAUREN HUTTON
2004 — MAGGIE GYLLENHAAL

# get the look

All-American sexy combines the best aspects of a uniform—a consistent look, fewer style dilemmas—without any actual combat requirement.

**This really is the simplest way** to live in clothes. Ask jeans-and-boots fan Cameron Diaz, who once went through a phase where she'd haul out the same outfit four days in a row. (Clearly, she wasn't in the mood to ponder fashion equations.) Or Jennifer Aniston: "Half the time," she's said, "I'll just pair a piece from my own closet, like an old T-shirt, with something like a fabulous pair of Gucci pants."

If you truly want to nail this style, however, you need to give it *some* thought. Remember, it took Jennifer years to distill her style from an unfocused twentysomething mess to the minimalist formula she's known for today. This isn't just Gap goes to the Oscars. There's a line between sloppy indifference and slouchy cool. Between plain and...beautifully plain.

**Fit and quality count big-time:** Like classic style, all-American sexy depends on simplicity. Neither look is big on pattern or design flourishes, so the fit of the individual pieces is crucial. "Comfort is always key," says celebrity stylist Jennifer Rade, who works with Angelina Jolie. "But at the same time, Angelina likes things that show off her body, just not in obvious ways."

Take the T-shirt, which Giorgio Armani has called the "alpha and omega of the fashion alphabet." To really work as a wardrobe player and not just something to nap in, a tee should meet certain fit and quality criteria:
- **Primo cotton:** A supple weight (medium thin, but not threadbare), 100-percent cotton (or with a bit of Lycra). Leave stiff, heavy cotton to the frat boys.
- **No flappy sleeves:** Choose more fitted

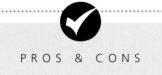

## PROS & CONS

### ALL-AMERICAN MAKES IT EASY

✳ **It puts comfort first:** You don't need to suffer for this art. No hobble skirts, no giant bows on your rear to make sitting a NASA-level challenge

✳ **It stays in style:** Remember the dorky tank tops of 1999? Of course not. Casual classics age better than "fashion." With updated accessories, you won't look stale.

✳ **It's quick:** Stick to mix-and-match separates, slip-on dresses, and anti wrinkle stretch fabrics, and you'll spend less time getting ready and more having fun.

### BUT WATCH OUT...

✳ **It's not particularly original:** This basics-heavy style can become predictable. When you want to stand out, push the color factor or use edgier jewelery.

✳ **It clashes with ladylike anything:** Don't try to daintify this strong look with proper handbags or kitten heels. Stick to bold or simply sexy accessories.

✳ **It's not perfect for every figure:** Skip the clingier knits and skimpier cuts if you're not so toned. A blazer and straight-leg pants, however, flatter almost anyone.

sleeves (or cap-sleeves for a feminine look).
- **A shape that's not too boxy or long:** Unless you're thinking minidress, a T-shirt really shouldn't fall past mid-hip.

Recently, Rade further refined the tee formula for Angelina. "Lately, I've been getting her T-shirts from C&C California with three-quarter sleeves and a wide boat neck, which widens your shoulders so your hips look smaller. And C&C's cotton is perfect—thin and soft."

Quality can cost, of course, but think of this like buying linens for your bed: You can sleep on the cheapest cotton, but if you spring for a higher thread count, it not only looks more beautiful, it's more sensual on the skin.

If your budget's tight, earmark a few investment pieces—a sharp suit, a silk (not acetate) skirt—to blow the bank on, or stalk until sale-time. Then back them up with good basics. And don't forget thrift stores, if you're willing to slog through racks of saggy, sandpapery polos that say "Applebee's" until fate reveals an Yves Saint Laurent silk shirt that truly needs rescuing.

**Build an army of separates:** There are plenty of dresses with an A.A. sexy vibe, but this look is anchored in interchangeable separates, elements that, in various combinations, can deliver both hanging-out and going-out looks. The jeans may get darker for night, the skirt shorter, the top more flowy. It's a fairly easy, low-stress approach.

But easy isn't automatically flattering, says Mary Alice Stephenson, who styles Liv Tyler. Wearing jeans with a top or a tank has

**Dress it up:** Statement accessories like **Mena Suvari**'s apple-green bag can push a primitive tank up the evolutionary scale.

**Add a jersey skirt:** "Extend" a black tank into a long sleek look. Curvier than **Selma Blair**? A flowy skirt works too.

# tank chic

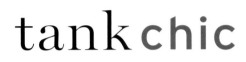

You can dress a tank top up, but you can't always take it out. A quick guide to the dos and dangers of wife-beater glam.

**Don't tart it up:** The laid-back factor eludes **Paris Hilton**. Our tips: Scrap the bow, get some flats, and learn to stand less thrustily.

**Don't go matronly:** Soccer mom or **Melissa Joan Hart**? Her tank's too long, cutting her at her thickest point, and its straps are too wide.

**Add a silky skirt:** **Jennifer Aniston** practically invented tank chic. She makes this one red-carpet ready by pairing it with an opulent Prada A-line skirt.

become a modern uniform, the ultimate no-brainer solution. "But ask yourself," says Stephenson, "Am I wearing this because everyone else is or because it looks good on me? Be honest about what works with your body." If you're pear-shaped, for instance, try switching in an A-line denim skirt and check out how that looks.

**Stick to basic solid colors:** The whole point of this style is to showcase *you*, not your clothes. Jennifer Aniston never wears technicolor or patterned pieces that compete for attention with her face or her hair. When you think of Jennifer, you think "healthy sexy" not "violet-and-peach corsety." **Most all-American:** All shades of brown (chocolate, chestnut, tan, camel), black, navy blue, khaki, cream, white. **Shake-it-up colors:** Red, green, orange, turquoise. **Avoid:** Pastels, fussy or overbearing prints.

**Mix in unique pieces:** When you're dressing in simple dresses or separates (especially if they're not especially deluxe), your look can seem generic. "Look for those special finds,"

---

ENTRY-LEVEL STYLE

## 10 EASY PIECES

Build the Jennifer Aniston look
one basic at a time

* Jeans in dark, unprocessed denim
* A sexy jersey dress
* A classic fitted blazer
* Refined high-heeled boots
* A silky, flowy skirt
* Sunglasses (dark as possible, with minimal glitz)
* Straight-leg tailored trousers
* Tank tops (white for day, black for night)
* A sleek black turtleneck
* Sandals (thong for day, simple and strappy for night)

---

says Rade, "like a great vintage camisole instead of a tank—pieces that are funky and cool and will work with the basics in your wardrobe." (She's boosted Angelina's stripped-down look with gold-embroidered capelets from Monique Lhuillier, for example.)

A pin-striped blazer from H&M can be a cheap fix, she says, even if the fit's a bit on the sloppy side: "Just pay a tailor $15 to have it nipped in at the waist."

**Remember, comfort can be sleek:** The wrap-dress has become a modern classic because of its body-conscious (but unconstricting) fit. "The wrap just works," says Stephenson. "The way it defines the waist and cups the breasts, but isn't so fitted around the thighs...and it's so comfortable." If you pay attention to fabric, says Rade, even something as potentially swamping as a poncho can be sexy: "You shouldn't wear a chunky cable-knit poncho unless you're 22 and Kate Hudson. I always choose thin cashmere, or superthin Iranian linen for Angelina, so you can still see her shape. It falls over the shoulder, and it's sexy without trying." Which is, of course, the ultimate goal.

### LABELS TO LOOK FOR

**Designer:** Michael Kors, Ralph Lauren, Calvin Klein, Giorgio Armani, Donna Karan
**More Affordable:** Kors by Michael Kors, Gap, Tommy Hilfiger, Diane Von Furstenberg, J.Crew

---

# ★ THE ALL-AMERICAN WRAP DRESS ★

Tie...and go. It may be the most universally flattering garment in history, and fuss-averse stars can't get enough of it.

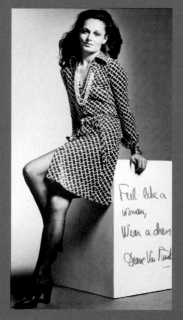

**In the early '70s,** the right to wear pants to work was considered a feminist victory, and women were making up for lost time. Then **Diane Von Furstenberg** (left) invented a zipperless dress that was just as straightforward but flattered curves in ways that made femininity hip again. By 1976, she was shipping 25,000 of her "wrap dresses" a week, and made *Newsweek*'s cover. Sales eventually dipped, but after a major revival in the late '90s, this slinky descendant of the kimono is here to stay.

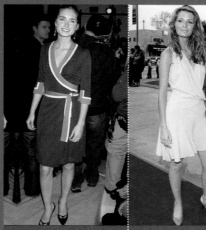

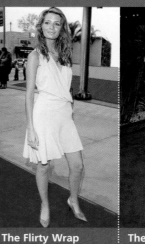

**The Classic Wrap**
**Lauren Bush** takes it easy in Diane Von Furstenburg's knit jersey, stripe-sashed version of her original straight-cut wrap.

**The Flirty Wrap**
**Mischa Barton**'s Plein Sud dress, a drapier cut flared to flutter and show off her stems, is not even slightly administrative.

**The Modern Wrap**
Loosely interpreting D.V.F.'s motto—"Feel like a woman, wear a dress!"—**Aisha Tyler** straps a mega-patterned wrap over jeans.

## Power Glam

The halter cut has a very American "athletic glamour," according to designer Marc Bouwer (a protégé of renowned '70s minimalist designer Halston). "A halter's long lines elongate the body, and make shoulders seem broader," adds Paul Margolin, president of Marc Bouwer. "You look taller, slimmer, yet powerful."

## Phantom Brooch

Rade considered adding a great piece of jewelry ("something with emeralds or rubies") in the center of the ruched "belt." In the end, the idea was scrapped to keep things even simpler.

## Red-Carpet Tats

"Angelina wanted 14-year-old girls to know you can have tattoos and still be totally glamorous," says Jolie's stylist Jennifer Rade. This tattoo, a Sanskrit prayer to protect Angelina's adopted son, Maddox, was reportedly applied by a Thai Buddhist monk using the traditional long-needles-and-hammer method, while she knelt with folded hands.

## Wrap as Bracelets

The two-foot-wide matching wrap, custom-made for Angelina, wasn't part of the runway version of the outfit. ("I kind of wish she hadn't worn it," Rade admits.) Bouwer gave her a little workshop on how to carry it lower on her wrists, so it didn't block the dress.

# ANATOMY OF
# A GOWN

**Angelina Jolie** *in Marc Bouwer at the 2004 Academy Awards: This halter dress may look simple, but it's actually a feat of bias-cut couture design.*

## As Seen on the Internet

Rade first spotted the gown on the Web, as part of Bouwer's 2004 fall collection. "It was beautifully simple," she says. "And not too cleavagey." The final choice came down to it and another Bouwer halter in black lace.

## Sneaky Artistry

Constructed of eight yards of heavy crepeback satin (most gowns average two to four yards), the gown achieves its mysterious rear swell via multiple panels, inserted using bias construction.

# Clean Finish

For all-American understatement, think hoop earrings, linear Jimmy Choos, and aviator sunglasses, the pinnacle of laid-back cool.

RAY-BAN AVIATORS Their history is macho: Originally designed in 1936 for air force pilots—who actually needed the sun's rays "banned" so they could stop squinting and efficiently bomb things—they've become the official antiglare shades of cops, truckers, and assorted Village People. Aviator shades can bestow on anyone, even the most uptight socialite, an air of "where would you like me to land this 747?" But if you wear them Jennifer Aniston–style, with sexy jeans, boots, and a sleek long-sleeved tee (braless if you're blessed with modest, '70s-style breasts), and stride across the first available wind-blown piazza, they can also just look…hot. If you can't find a piazza, pretty much any old street will do.

### textured clutch
No glitz—just subtle graphic quilting

FRANCHI

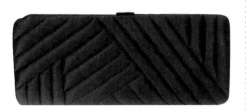

### minimalist earrings
360 degrees of chic

JULIE SANDLAU

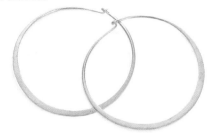

### sinuous sandals
Unembellished strappiness

JIMMY CHOO

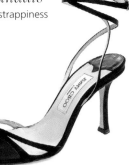

### roll bag
As compact as minidachsund, but less yappy

MICHAEL BY MICHAEL KORS

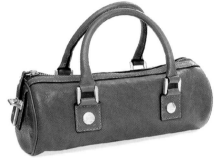

### power bracelet
A '70s classic: Elsa Peretti's sculptured silver cuff

ELSA PERETTI AT TIFFANY & CO.

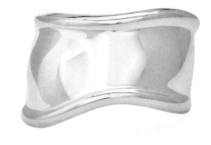

### strong boots
Low-key design is key.

MARC JACOBS

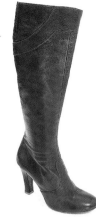

## unfinicky bags

## bold strokes

## pure footwear

### american classic
The saddle bag, once reserved for horses

CHLOE

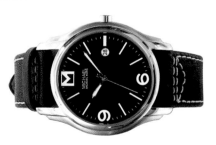

### men's-style watch
No gimmicks: You're not interested in tricks of the wrist.

MICHAEL BY MICHAEL KORS

### chic loafers
Elegant shape meets all-American color

TODS

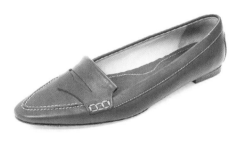

### luxe tote
Simple, capacious, suede

BALLY

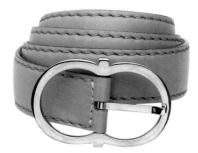

### unbasic belt
A restrained but highly distinctive buckle

SALVATORE FERRAGAMO

### bare necessity
The perfect thong, neither too fancy nor beachy

BERNARDO

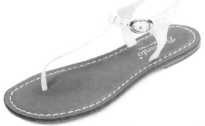

# chapter 5

# ULTRA-GLAM

If you're a shy soul who loves a cozy Fair Isle sweater, turn back now. Ultra-glam women like **Beyoncé** and **Jennifer Lopez** come from a different isle. They don't expect clothing to be sensible. Or especially comfortable. (You don't need "cozy" to make an entrance.) They value the hard work of corsets, and rank stilettos as a necessity. Even if they owned no clothes, they'd figure out a way to wear large leaves with a deadly bravado. That confidence is key: When you're too embarrassed to pull off crystal beading, when you slouch and roll your eyes and make it seem like a chore, you're not glamorous. (You're just a sloucher littered with shiny bits.) Like love, glamour only happens when you truly commit—if not 24/7, then at least for one amazing night.

"I want to be a legend."

—BEYONCÉ KNOWLES

# Charlize Theron

Though more of a jeans girl off-duty, she's perfected a **turbocharged elegance** for the red carpet that's pure movie star.

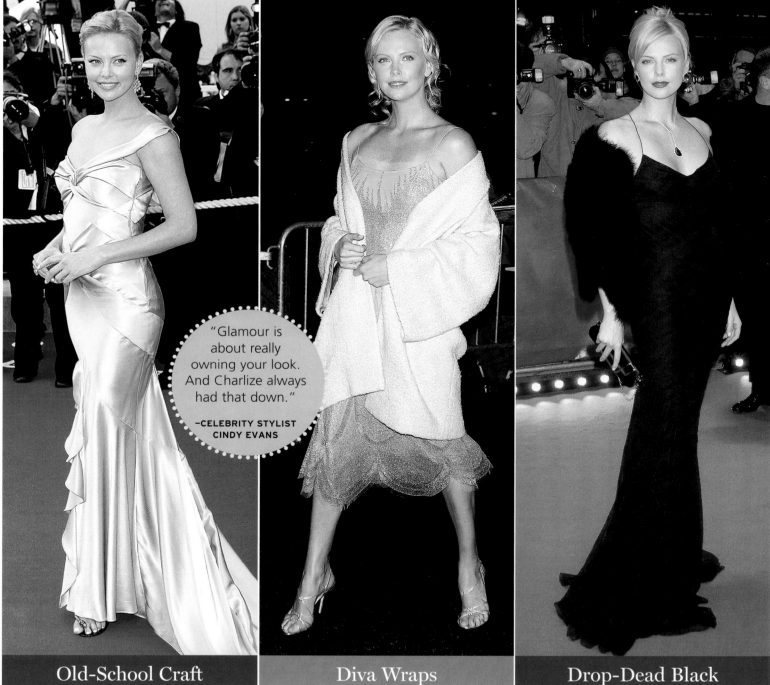

"Glamour is about really owning your look. And Charlize always had that down."

**—CELEBRITY STYLIST CINDY EVANS**

## Old-School Craft

As intricate as origami, this Christian Dior gown is bias-cut. (The fabric was cut diagonally across the weave, which helps it drape and hug the body more sensually.)

## Diva Wraps

The key move here is the way Charlize lets her sumptuous wrap fall off her shoulders. It just isn't glamorous to make your big arrival all sensibly bundled up.

## Drop-Dead Black

Ultra-glam style isn't especially "nice." Black, often merely chic, becomes darkly seductive with a gown that fits as wickedly as this spaghetti-strapped Christian Dior slip dress.

# Halle Berry

Her take is more ornate, but not at the expense of sexy—and she's often worn her hair cropped to give glamour **an anti-Barbie Doll twist.**

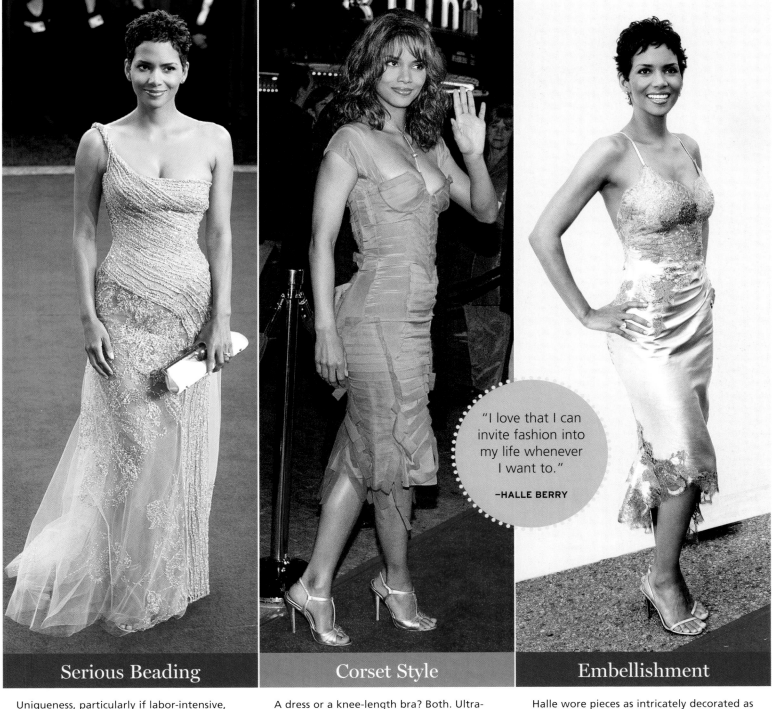

> "I love that I can invite fashion into my life whenever I want to."
>
> **—HALLE BERRY**

### Serious Beading

### Corset Style

### Embellishment

Uniqueness, particularly if labor-intensive, is a big part of glamour. It can take weeks to hand-bead a masterwork like Halle's asymmetrical Elie Saab gown, and it shows.

A dress or a knee-length bra? Both. Ultra-glam women, never timid when it comes to sexiness, love body-conscious styles like this Dolce & Gabbana corset number.

Halle wore pieces as intricately decorated as this 2002 lace-appliqué slip dress well before sequined-and-embroidered-everything became a broader fashion trend.

# Jennifer Lopez

Jennifer is the essence of **shameless, full-throttle glamour:** Has she ever betrayed the slightest hint of self-consciousness?

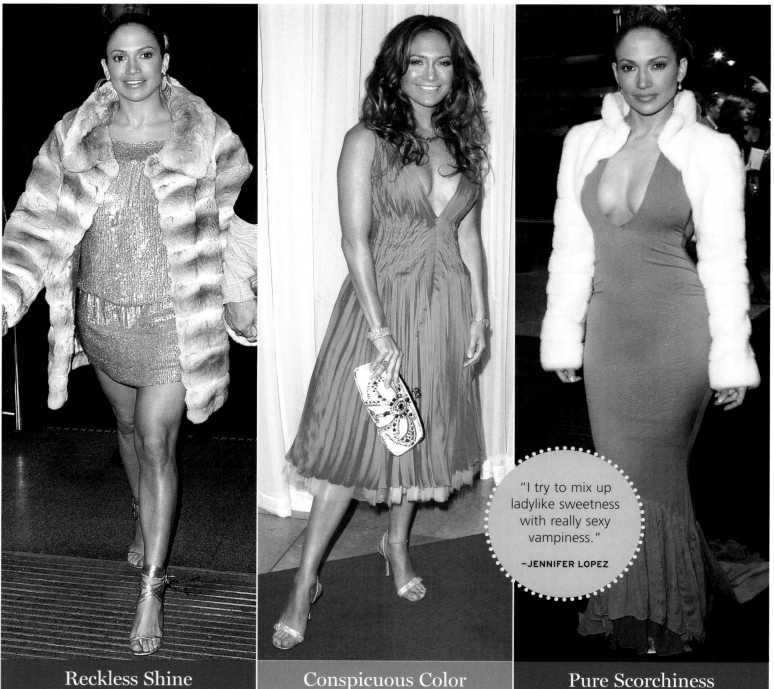

"I try to mix up ladylike sweetness with really sexy vampiness."

–JENNIFER LOPEZ

### Reckless Shine

### Conspicuous Color

### Pure Scorchiness

The unglamorous are matte. The glamorous frequently shine. Here, J. Lo approximates a 19,000-carat diamond thanks to a sequined minidress, gilded sandals, and body shimmer.

Glamour needs to be noticed, or it can't do its job. Jennifer works a J. Mendel dress in a fairly riveting shade of coral. A gauzey underskirt adds a gentler note.

A very committed J. Lo mermaids herself inside a hobble-skirt gown—*you* try walking in one—then dramatically frames her cleavage with a Fendi fur bolero jacket.

# [DENIM GLAM]

*To truly diva-fy jeans these days, you need more than a cute top. You need a stupendous top. Ditto jacket. Ditto purse.*

*Giant satin-lined cuffs*

*Major chandelier earrings*

*Retro-'70s patch-pocket jeans*

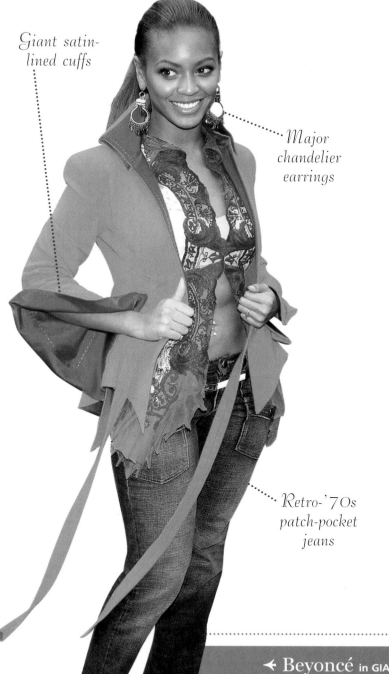

### Uma Thurman ➤
**with a LOUIS VUITTON bag**
Even laid-back glamour has to be balanced. This wouldn't work as well if Uma didn't have the gold status bag to offset the mammoth flower. And vice versa.

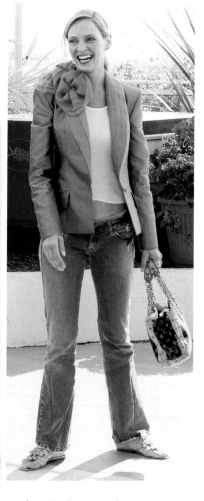

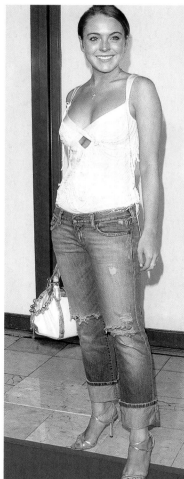

### ◀ Lindsay Lohan
**in a TOP-TO-END-ALL-TOPS**
Denim glam is the ultimate mix of the raw and the ornate. Lindsay contrasts ratty jeans with a masterpiece of cute-toppiness that festoons her bosom with dozens of silky cords.

### ◀ Beyoncé in GIANFRANCO FERRÉ
The child of destiny goes over the top in a Ferré top and jacket so fierily flamboyant they threaten to inflame her jeans. Notice how unconcerned she appears? That's glamour.

# MARILYN MONROE

## Patron Saint of Style

····················· Supershine ·····················

**Then:** Marilyn in the controversial gold-lamé dress from *Gentlemen Prefer Blondes* (in which it's briefly shown from behind) that nearly ruined her career. **Now:** Kim Cattrall and Beyoncé, both wearing Carmen Marc Valvo.

····················· Bouffants ·····················

**Then:** Marilyn's hair got bigger and blonder in the '60s as she drifted into self-parody. **Now:** Jessica Simpson, another knowingly "dumb" blonde, tries the style on for size.

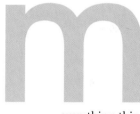

marilyn Monroe's closet was often nearly empty. In 1954, she owned little except a few undistinguished sweaters, a mink coat, and some tight cropped pants. No Balenciaga. No Christian Dior. Almost everything this future pop-culture icon wore—even just to hit a restaurant—was borrowed for the day or the weekend from her movie studio's wardrobe department, and designed by its costumers (primarily William Travilla). For Monroe, being "Marilyn" was as much a role as any of her onscreen characters, which says a lot about glamour. These loaner clothes weren't pieces she treasured, just tools to help her turn her image on and off. ("It's no fun being married to an electric light," beefed her second husband, Joe DiMaggio.)

Sometimes she dangerously blurred the lines between fantasy and reality. When she needed a suitable dress for the 1953 Photoplay Awards, she ignored everyone's advice and wore a skintight gold-lamé gown from her

## Starburst Pleats

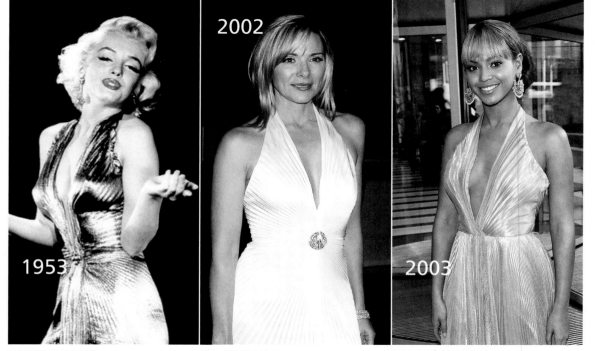

1953 — MARILYN MONROE
2002 — KIM CATTRALL
2003 — BEYONCÉ KNOWLES

## Big Blondes

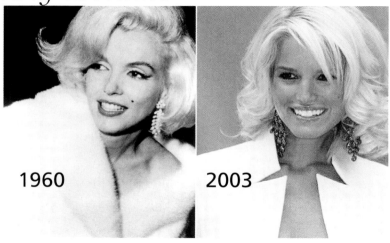

1960 — MARILYN MONROE
2003 — JESSICA SIMPSON

*Gentlemen Prefer Blondes* wardrobe. On camera, its tissue-thin fabric seemed more substantial, but in real life, according to witnesses, she looked vulgarly naked. Her arrival provoked jeers and laughter (shades of Paris Hilton), and a national uproar led by Joan Crawford, but the success of *Blondes* shut everyone up.

Marilyn, an orphan who was named Miss California Artichoke in 1947, may not have had the unerring fashion instincts of a Jackie Kennedy, but both women understood the gospel of glamour: The right clothing matters, but bravado is crucial. And that's how, at least for a while, Marilyn overcame her humble roots and her lethal insecurities. "I used to say to myself," she once admitted. "'What the devil have you got to be proud about, Marilyn Monroe?' And I'd answer, 'Everything, *everything*,' and I'd walk slowly and turn my head slowly, as if I were a queen."

# get the look

It's easier than ever to dress "glamorously," but true glamour is not just about glitz. It's really a way of thinking.

**Most of us don't spend a lot of time** in gowns. They're really not that practical for the subway, and bosses tend to fire women who drag 4-foot satin trains down the hall to the photocopier. So let's forget about gowns for the moment. And feather boas, and long silk gloves, and all the other Boris-and-Natasha clichés the word "glamour" conjures up.

Glamour can be as simple as red lipstick. Or as private as a tangerine silk lining inside a tweed jacket. Even with the growing army of sequined tops out there, you can't just pick it up at the mall. The truth, says stylist Rachel Zoe Rosenzweig, who's worked with Jennifer Garner and Jessica Simpson, is that clothing (not to mention hair and makeup) is only part of the equation; the rest is attitude.

**It starts with you:** "Anybody can be glamorous," says Rosenzweig. "In Hollywood, you see so many transformations, actresses who go from the worst-dressed lists to fashion-icon status. It happens when they finally say, I care now and I want people to look at me and go, 'Wow!' " Ego has always fueled fashion; few people dress up to be ignored. So if you think it's somehow wrong to do your bit to increase the world's supply of glamour, this isn't going to work. "You have to be into it," says George Blodwell, who's styled the generally enthusiastic Drew Barrymore. "I always find happy women the most glamorous."

Tap into the guilt-free pleasures of playing dress-up as a kid. (Cate Blanchett used to let her sister costume her, then Cate would stay

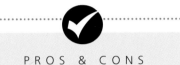

## PROS & CONS

### ULTRA-GLAM GETS YOU NOTICED

❋ **It catches the eye:** Anything shiny, from a metallic belt to a sequined top, lowers the risk of being rudely ignored at parties. Or hockey games.

❋ **It welcomes curves:** With luscious, form-fitting clothes, a voluptuous figure is often an advantage. No one wants to see bones in a corset.

❋ **It's expressive:** Unlike monks, who have little to work with (brown burlap and rope), you've got crystals, beads, metallics, fur, the list goes on...

### BUT WATCH OUT...

❋ **It's not always appropriate:** Glam is not suitable for funerals, protests, or giving birth, but usually, it's a question of how much, not all-or-nothing.

❋ **Other women might resent you:** A smile always helps (who resents Kate Hudson?), but envy comes with the territory. Rise above it, in stilettos.

❋ **It's not always big on comfort:** If you're not one of those "Actually, I'm more comfortable in heels" women, this may not be your look.

in character for days.) Put on something that's bright, shiny, sexy, or luxurious enough to nudge you out of your everyday existence, then go out in public. Imagine that it's truly your duty to enliven the crowd's dull existence. (Admittedly tricky in rural areas.) Once you tap into the attitude, the clothes matter less. "Sometimes I feel glamorous even when I'm not put together," says Eve's personal stylist Erin Hirsh. "I have this child-size blue hoodie sweatshirt that's been through everything. But if my hair and makeup are right, and I've thrown on some dressy shoes, even that sweatshirt can be glamorous."

**A little glitz can certainly help:** Thanks to fashion's recent obsession with embellishment, there's been no shortage of options. (Even preppy J.Crew has sold sequined camisoles.) Focus on real wardrobe builders: A brocade skirt, some crystal-sparked heels, a beaded halter-top. (If you're not ready for J. Lo–level shine, tone down a glitzy piece with something quieter; a cashmere sweater can hush a silver skirt nicely.) Rosenzweig prefers crystals to sequins: "It's a richer look, and it picks up the light better. Sequins can easily go bad '80s prom." For her part, Hirsh is looking for alternatives to glitter: "The question always becomes 'what's next?' At the moment, I'm intrigued by pieces with unusual kinds of leather trim."

**Think beyond the surface:** Let the sequins fall as they may. Fit and fabric will always

# 5

## levels of embellishment

**Choose your shine strategy:** Glow in plain silk, sparkle slightly, or light up the entire room. (Helpful for anyone trying to read.)

## 1. unadorned

**[SCA]RLETT [JOH]ANSSON** in [Ca]lvin Klein [Som]etimes it's [best] to let silk do [the jo]b alone. It's [amply] qualified.

## 2. beaded details

**KATIE HOLMES in Carolina Herrera** Discreet glitz, like this lightly beaded bodice, is ideal for the glamour girl-next-door.

## 3. glam collage

**[MILL]A JOVOVICH** [in Pr]ada [For a] mid-level [look], mix silk [and] sequins [(in on]e dress [or by] pairing [separ]ates).

## 4. major shine

**MISCHA BARTON in Maggie Norris Couture** In a fully beaded dress, you need to radiate, too, or risk being overshadowed.

## 5. maxed-out

**CHLOE SEVIGNY in Oscar de la Renta** Feathers, sequins, ruffles, bows... sometimes excess is a mess, but here it works.

### The Concept

A modern, unstructured version of Marilyn Monroe's famous "nude" dresses. "Charlize liked the idea of a simple slip dress that hangs off the body delicately," says Evans, "as opposed to something cinched in and corseted and over-the-top." Result: an unusually comfortable couture gown.

### Golden Girl

Makeup artist Shane Paish used body bronzer, "so that Charlize's skin would really pop against the flesh-colored dress." He may have overachieved. "She wasn't meant to be quite so golden," laughs stylist Cindy Evans, who's spent a lot of time explaining that no spray-tan misadventures were involved: "Charlize was already super tan from a vacation in Brazil."

### Fitting Fix

When the gown, as originally conceived, proved too unstructured and loose, Gucci creative director David Bamber improvised this extra strap to cup the bust and wrap tightly around the back.

### Snip Before Bed

Charlize was sewn into the gown on Oscar day, but Bamber left her a little pair of scissors, so she could liberate herself at the end of a long night.

# ANATOMY OF
# A GOWN

*Charlize Theron* in Tom Ford for Gucci at the 2004 Academy Awards: She wanted to avoid making a "huge statement" by opting for a low-key slip dress. Nice try.

### Confetti

Crystal beading, dense at the bodice, grows sparser toward the hem. The Gucci design team "wanted a feeling that the crystals had been thrown over Charlize like confetti, so that when she moved there would be an intense sparkle around her face."

### Where Is It Now?

"Charlize gets her gowns cleaned, then preserved in a private storage space in special acid-free boxes," says Evans. "These dresses really are masterpieces."

# Added Attractions

Triple the allure with accessories no one could possibly overlook. A diamond (or 192) is always a nice touch.

ROCK STARS Diamond jewelry—like this 40-carat necklace we borrowed, nervously, from Harry Winston—epitomizes glamour. Just ask poor Minnie Driver, who ended up crawling awkwardly around the red carpet at the 1998 Oscars, desperately trying to find the rocks that went AWOL after her diamond bracelet broke. (She recovered all but one.) Diamonds didn't always cause such a fuss: Before the Academy Awards were first televised in 1953, those stars who even aspired to high glamour (unlike Ingrid Bergman, who wore the same drab black dress two years running) favored pearls. These days, Los Angeles–based jeweler Martin Katz has said, the hunt for the perfect Oscar diamonds has become so competitive that certain A-list actresses and their stylists borrow the best pieces and then hoard them until the big night has passed, ensuring they'll outshine their rivals. You'd never do that...would you?

### royal-jewel clutch
Tastefully extravagant, with a retro closure
CHLOÉ

### cocktail rings
Affordable flash—and almost as big as ice-cubes
RJ GRAZIANO

### t-strap heels
The straps should be as thin as possible.
POLLINI

### satin poof
A girlier take on evening glamour
KATE SPADE

### chandelier earrings
The more elaborate, the better
ERICKSON BEAMON

### bouclé pumps
Lavish textures fit your style.
MOSCHINO

# luxe bags

# glam boosters

# showy shoes

### envy-provoking purse
Appropriately green
JIMMY CHOO

### suede gloves
In impractical pink
VALENTINO

### minx mules
To be kicked off in moments of kittenish zeal
BRIAN ATWOOD

### chic tote
Ooh la la large
POLLINI

### extreme shades
Either pitch-black or pointlessly pale. Nothing in between
VALENTINO

### beaded flats
As close to "casual" as Ultra-Glam gets
GINA

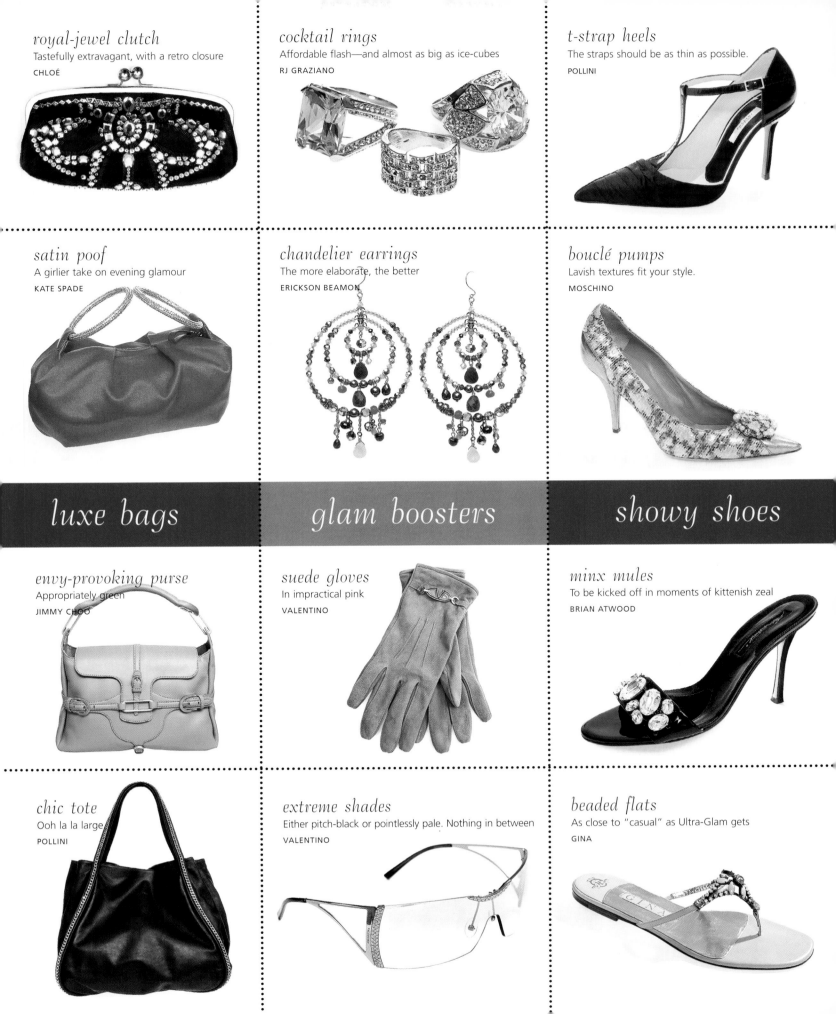

# "I'M SAD TO SAY THAT MY MULLET IS GONE."

—SCARLETT JOHANSSON ON HER CONVERSION TO GLAMOUR

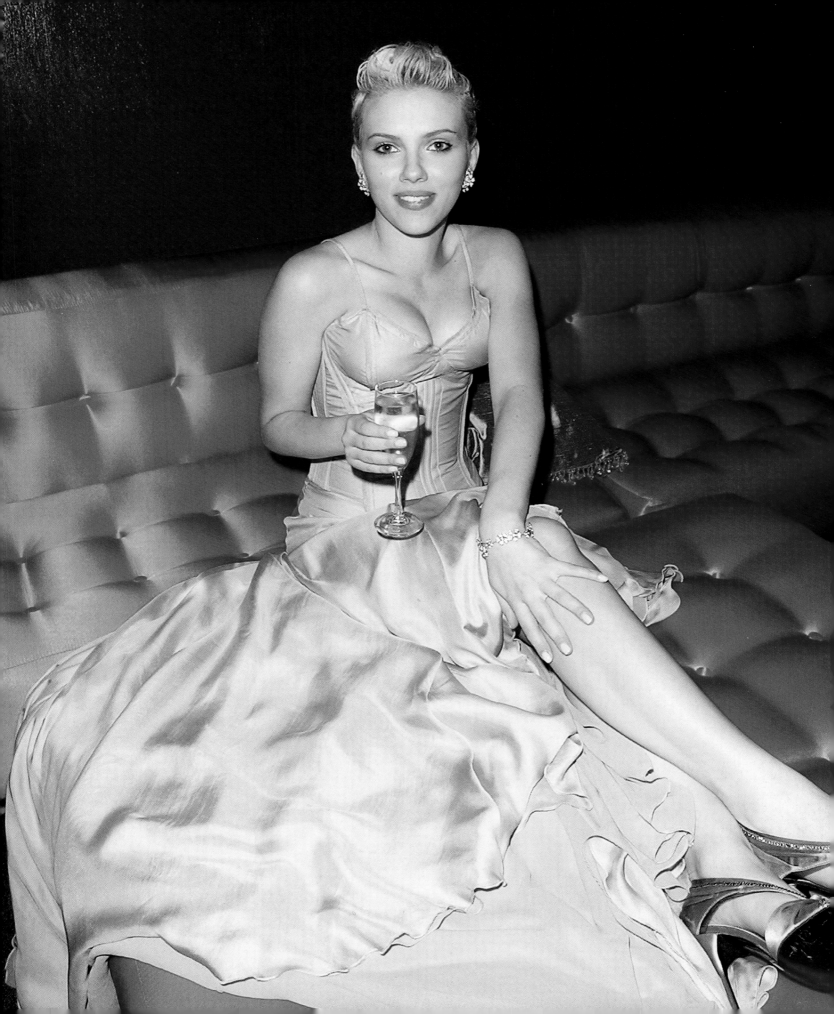

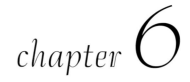

# CHAMELEON

There's only one thing consistent about chameleon style: a wonderful lack of consistency.

Like the little lizard for which this strategy is named, chameleons such as **Uma Thurman** and **Mandy Moore** regularly change their look depending on the occasion or their whims. (Of course, Uma and Mandy are considerably leggier than the lizard and eat far fewer fruit flies.) Chameleons will choose a classic Chanel suit when demure is called for, or conjure up a creative get-up when ignoring fashion rules feels right. They keep people guessing ("What will she show up in this time?") and dabble in a variety of mood-altering jeans. If this is your style, you want that versatility, the freedom to work almost any look—even if it requires a much bigger closet.

# Uma Thurman

As Uma once summed up **her style philosophy**: "When everyone looks the same in their spaghetti-strapped, sequined, chiffon things...you get bored."

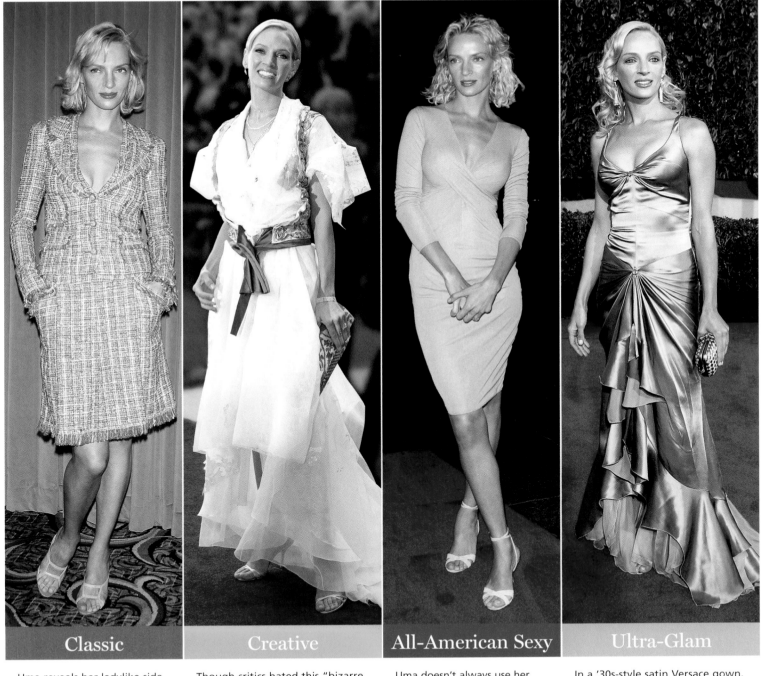

| Classic | Creative | All-American Sexy | Ultra-Glam |
|---|---|---|---|
| Uma reveals her ladylike side (and some serious cleavage) in a proper Chanel suit that's mildly unhinged with fringe. | Though critics hated this "bizarre flamenco-milkmaid" creation by Christian Lacroix, it showcases Uma's who-cares versatility. | Uma doesn't always use her killer body, but it's hard to miss in this lilac bodyglove (worn with minimal jewelry). | In a '30s-style satin Versace gown, Uma proves she can outglam them all if necessary. Best feature: the frothy peekaboo underskirt. |

# Garcelle Beauvais-Nilon

**A pro at dressing for occasions**, this impossible-to-pigeonhole star always looks turned out, no matter what she turns up in.

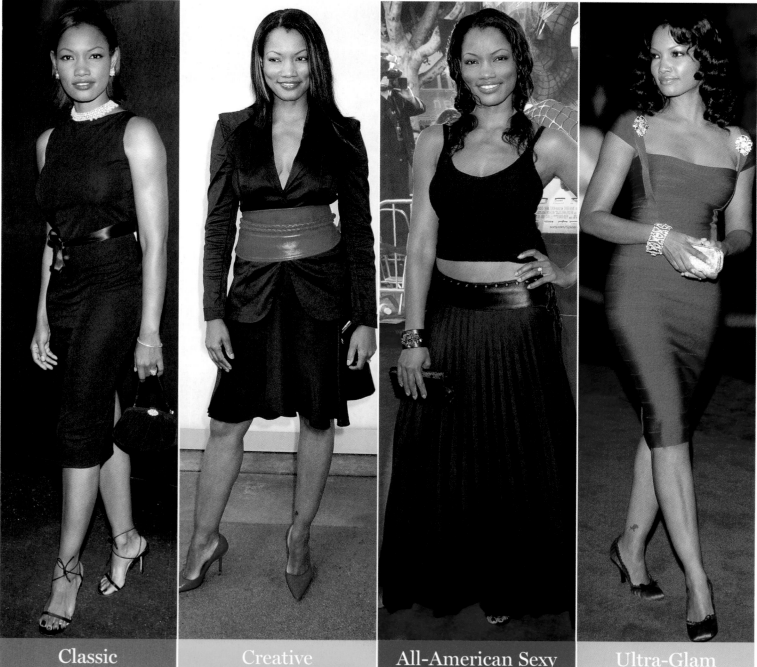

**Classic**

**Creative**

**All-American Sexy**

**Ultra-Glam**

Garcelle successfully combines sexy and formal in a slinky Mark Zuzino socialite sheath, dignified with a pearl choker.

In theory, the idea of cinching a Fendi blazer with a red leather cummerbund sounds terrible. In practice, it kinda rocks.

For a summer premiere, Garcelle chills a long pleated skirt with a tank (but keeps both pieces black for sophistication).

In a very "movie star" Hervé Leger dress, Garcelle ups the glam with not one, but two supernova brooches.

# Mandy Moore

We freely admit it—we love this girl. Just look at her: never costumey, always cool, and **effortlessly versatile**.

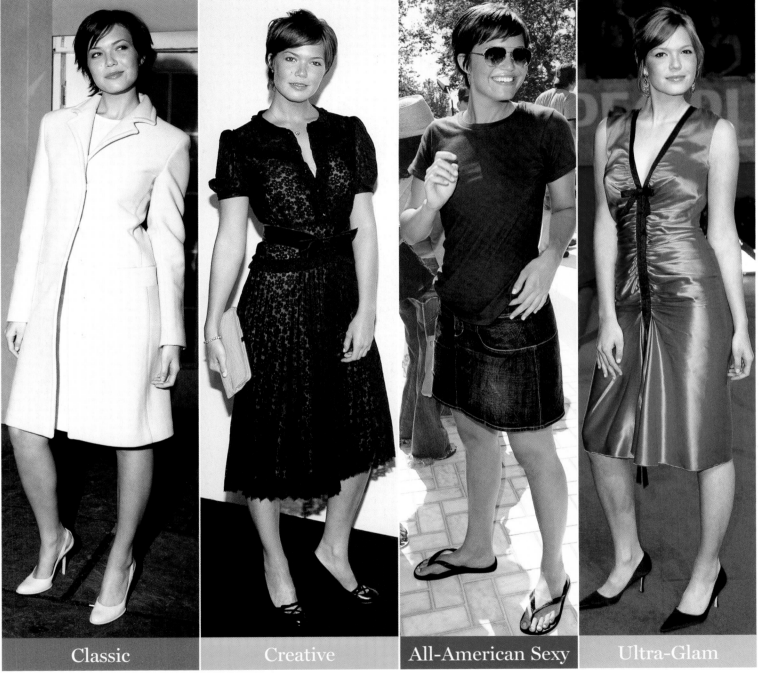

| Classic | Creative | All-American Sexy | Ultra-Glam |

Mandy goes the traditional route in a tailored coat by Narciso Rodriguez with Jackie Kennedy's signature lapel edging.

The genius stroke here is the shock of the yellow clutch, which gives Mandy's polite Marc Jacobs dress a bit of '80s brattiness.

Taking it easy in a perfectly cut tee and a cute, nongimmicky jean skirt. Her aviator sunglasses say, "No stress here, man."

Too young for an old-school gowny gown, Mandy works a ruched Lanvin dress that's modern but still grand.

# The Little Black Chameleon

Attention restless cocktail partiers! A change of accessories can give a little black dress a whole new persona.

*classic*
ELEGANT

*creative*
MADCAP

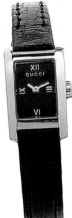

❋ **Send a plain black sheath dress** to finishing school by upping its essential sophistication with low-key accessories: A **Gucci** tank watch, a proper structured bag, satin mules (very **Catherine Zeta-Jones**), and pearl earrings that evoke a witty Vassar grad in 1961. Or 2005.

❋ **The same black dress gets capricious** and impatient to dance with vintage-inspired accessories: flirty **Milla Jovovich**-ish stilettos, a swingy necklace looped twice flapper-style, and a beaded bag calculated to catch the light. For those who want to look more literally madcap: a '20s-style cloche hat with its own brooch.

> "Brighter, busier clothing can dictate a woman's mood and her actions. A little black dress never overpowers; it allows a woman to play a whole range of parts."
>
> —LEGENDARY FASHION EDITOR GRACE CODDINGTON

*all-american sexy*
STRAIGHTFORWARD

*ultra-glam*
DIVA

✳ **The L.B.D. becomes simply chic** in that **Jennifer Aniston** way when you play it down with minimalist, sculptural extras: a men's-style **Rolex** watch, glossy black boots, a half-moon clutch, and silver drop earrings as purely geometric as prisms.

✳ **With some glitzy additions,** the modest sheath is quite prepared to take over the world: bag and shoes by **Valentino**, a fur shrug fastened with an art-deco pin, star-shaped earrings, and—think **J. Lo**—elbow-length gloves. **For full fashion credits, see page 221.**

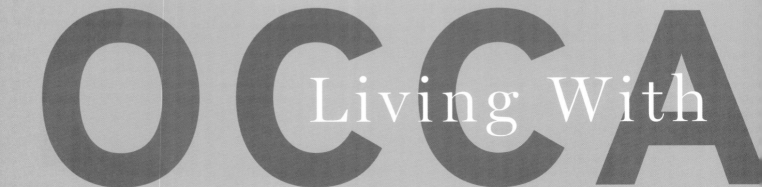

# PART THREE

OCCA

Living With

**Whether Gwyneth Paltrow's out** picking up groceries or collecting an Oscar, there's something fundamentally Gwyneth about her style. She doesn't think in terms of "everyday me" and "going-out me." She just adapts her look to whatever's going on. As you develop your own signature style, that flexibility is the goal. For those dozing-on-the-sofa moments, anything's appropriate, but for your more public appearances—from a casual date to a formal wedding—it's worth checking out how celebrities in the four main style categories shift their look up or down.

SIONS

Celebrity Style

# chapter 7

# DAYTIME

You see celebrities in so many evening gowns, it's easy to assume they only come out at night, like unusually glamorous bats. Not true. In their daylight hours, they have children to push on swings, overpriced lattes to buy, agents to fire over lunch at the Ivy in Santa Monica. And, like most off-duty women, they get tempted by shlubbiness—you might recall the extended love affair Jennifer Aniston conducted a few years ago with a certain pair of rumpled orange Maharishi cargo pants. Other stars, such as hippie-chic **Kate Hudson** or the tirelessly stylish **Selma Blair**, rarely indulge in such frumpy comfort. And when you're strategizing daytime outfits for a date, a brunch, a wedding, their looks tend to be a lot more inspiring than Jennifer's oh-so-relatable, yet regrettable, orange pants.

"If I feel good in something—like I could run a marathon in it—I'll wear it."

—KATE HUDSON

# shopping

**The number one rule of shopping style:** dress up a little and you'll get better service—at least until Penélope Cruz strolls in.

**We've all experienced that soul-sucking moment** of Being Totally Ignored in some boutique—just because you happen to be wearing your cool but ratty Earth Day T-shirt. "It's terrible, but it happens," says **Tracey Ross**, whose Los Angeles store, Tracey Ross, is a favorite pit stop for stars like **Charlize Theron** and **Selma Blair**. ("They know they can come through the back door before we open," she says, "with no makeup, and not have to worry about being 'on.'") If rattiness can make you ignorable, however, overdressing can make you look insecure. Even though Ross's store is unusually welcoming, her nonfamous customers often try too hard to impress: "They come in with their status Prada bags and their Bulgari watches," she says. "Personally, I'd rather see someone who just has a really good vibe, a personal style." Bonus budget benefit: When you know you're looking chic, it's easier to avoid that reckless "I'm a slob, I better buy a whole new wardrobe right now!" reaction. Other strategies:

✳ **DRESS FOR EFFICIENCY:** If you're trying on a lot, wear slip-off shoes and loose tops you can pull over your head.

✳ **USE SHORTCUTS:** Wear an A-line skirt if you want to test pants quickly and skip dressing-room lines.

✳ **ALWAYS CARRY AS LITTLE AS POSSIBLE:** No dry-cleaning bags, no books, no Chihuahuas.

## Classic

**PENÉLOPE CRUZ in nautical chic:**
Without that jumbo bow, this navy-blue top and white jeans combo would be natty but routine. In true classic style, the bow is the sole flourish—Penélope's matching tote and shoes have only low-key details

### Dress Whites
A nautical color scheme is one of the few situations in which white shoes don't look lame (unless you think nautical color schemes *themselves* are lame).

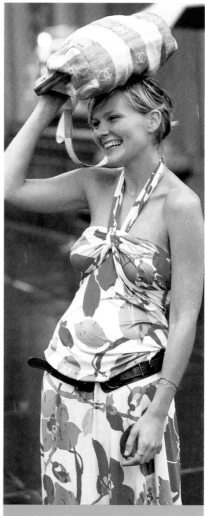

### Creative

**KIRSTEN DUNST works a hipster-goes-Bahamas look:** "There's a difference between dressing-down cool and not so cool," says Ross. Walk into a store in a tropical sundress expertly de-cheesed with a tough leather belt —and they'll know you're no ordinary shopper. Another clue: the many, many Chanel logos on your purse.

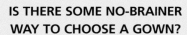

### Q.

### IS THERE SOME NO-BRAINER WAY TO CHOOSE A GOWN?

In a word, no. Stylist **Rachel Zoe Rosenzweig**, who's made some stars try on more than 30 gowns to find the right one, breaks it down:

✳ **Don't overlook that sparkly sock:** "Try on as much as possible to see what works on your body. It might look like a sock with sparkles on the hanger, and then you put it on, and...wow."

✳ **Ignore trends:** "Don't follow fashion, follow your body. And when in doubt, go simple. Women try to push it and they end up going over the top."

✳ **Beware cruel fabrics:** "Silk charmeuse is glamorous, but clingy. If you're insecure about your body, try a heavier jersey, taffeta, or duchesse satin."

✳ **Bring a trusted advisor:** "But ignore her if she says you look really skinny or hot in a gown you don't feel comfortable in. You won't wear it well."

matter more than decorative trends, says Blodwell, especially when it comes to that special-occasion gown: "Dressing a star is not really about fashion. It's about how the gown will work on camera. It has to show the lines of the body, and it can't make her look too big." The goal is a confident, knowing sexiness, which often means a body-hugging fit and a pair of Spanx, the "power panties" beloved by celebrities. As Rosenzweig points out, it helps if there's a body to hug, ideally a fairly voluptuous one: "It's actually hard to be glamorous if you're a size zero skeleton."

Whatever your body type, make sure you don't ignore fabric. "You want one with enough weight to hang and not just cling," says Hirsh. "I don't get the popularity of Viscose, for instance—it shows every flaw."

**Think beyond the obvious:** Shine helps, sexy tailoring helps. But as anyone who's seen the famous photos of Marilyn Monroe laughing on the beach in a big sweater (and little else) knows, glamour doesn't need to be elaborate. It can be as quick as a tiny chiffon scarf tied around your neck, à la Natalie Wood. If you're unfamiliar with Natalie, Google her.

Or rent *Splendor in the Grass* on DVD. The wider your frame of reference, the less predictable your take on glamour will be.

**A word about comfort:** Ouch. The ultra-glam style, with its corsets and potentially scratchy beads, often has little in common with a nice hot bath. Eve once raced another woman in stilettos and won, but if that's not you, find a less elevated route to glamour, or take precautions. (Stylists swear by Foot Petals cushions, created for women with "a love/hate relationship" with sexy shoes.) Then again, says Angelina Jolie's stylist Jennifer Rade (who is pro-corset as long as the boning is flexible plastic), "Comfort is partly mental. You're willing to put up with a fair bit if you look really good. It's like there's comfort, and then there's comforting. If you know you have this sexy, womanly shape, that's very comforting."

#### LABELS TO LOOK FOR

**Designer:** Versace, Dolce & Gabbana, Valentino, Oscar de la Renta, Rochas, Christian Lacroix
**Affordable:** Karl Lagerfeld for H&M, BCBG Max Azria, Bebe, Banana Republic

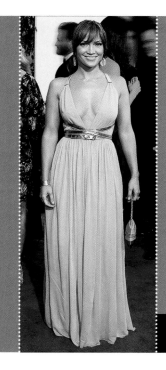

## LOOKALIKE GLAM

Thanks to ABS by Allen Schwartz and the red-carpet clone industry, you can literally dress like the stars.

Each year, as the Oscar telecast yawns to a close, the folks at ABS by Allen Schwartz are already stitching up their knockoffs of the stars' gowns. By 6 A.M., in some cases, they've finished their interpretations—simplified, sometimes recast in more palatable colors, and ready to rush into production. Are the ABS versions worth their $300-plus prices? "I'd always rather see people interpret a look their own way rather than copy it," says stylist Rachel Zoe Rosenzweig, "but I think ABS is a good alternative for women without $20,000 to spare on couture. Obviously, the craftsmanship and fabric aren't even close, but how many people are going to come up to your gown and touch it?" Not counting creepy people, that is.

**HEY, THAT'S MY DRESS:** J. Lo's Michael Kors (left) and ABS's version (right).

> "Women dress up to go shopping because it makes them feel more confident—more like part of the gang. Everyone wants to get noticed. "
>
> —**TRACEY ROSS**, OWNER OF THE CELEB-MAGNET L.A. BOUTIQUE TRACEY ROSS

**STYLIST TIP:**
Always take a pair of heels along if you're shopping for clothes that need them.

## All-American Sexy

**UMA THURMAN revs up basics:** Not much obvious "fashion" here. But Uma's hip flats and shades—not to mention a sharp eye for proportions—turn this into a take-me-seriously outfit. (A longer tank would have made her tiny jean jacket look *too* dwarfy.)

## Ultra-Glam

**KATE MOSS in laid-back fur:** The most glamorous thing about this look is the casual way that Kate has slipped her fur jacket over a droopy cowl-necked sweatshirt and jeans. The mix says "assured style-setter," instead of "clueless rich bitch."

# big-deal brunch

Whether it's your mom's birthday brunch or your competitive friend's annual "Bellinis 'n' Waffles" event, **leave your jeans at home.**

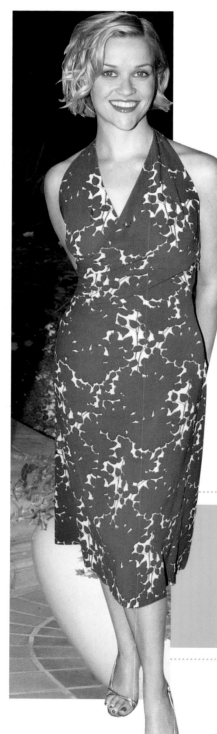

**"Stars have to dress up constantly,"** says stylist Danna Weiss, who helps **Molly Sims** keep up with the cycle. "But mere mortals have far fewer occasions to get really dressed." One exception? The special-occasion brunch. (As opposed to the hungover brunch where the key challenge is remembering to wear actual clothes, not pajamas.) "With the whole ladylike trend," says Tamara Rappa, a New-York–based stylist who's worked with **Scarlett Johansson**, "women have begun to wear denim less and less for occasions. The dress has definitely made a comeback." How to make sure you're not trying *too* hard:

✳ DON'T SHOW UP IN A FITTED SATIN SHEATH: "Stiff shiny fabrics just aren't appropriate for day," says Rappa. Think cotton voile, silk georgette, chiffon, lightweight knits, or if you're feeling Swiss, eyelet.

✳ WORK WITH EMBELLISHED SEPARATES: A dress isn't the only option. The recent ardor for ornament has made it easy to find casual yet dressy separates: beaded cardigans, ribbon-trimmed blazers, embroidered silk tops. "Wear one classic piece with fancy details," says Rappa, "and then calm it down with something more casual, like a cotton skirt."

✳ AVOID UPTIGHT SHOES: Closed-toe pumps can look too formal for brunch. Show some ground-level skin in peep-toe shoes, delicate sandals, or flats perforated with interesting cut-outs.

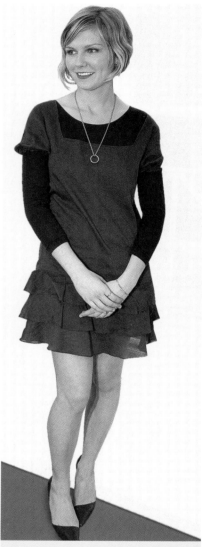

## Classic

**REESE WITHERSPOON in ladylike Prada:** With its minty, leafy print, this feminine dress (ideally cut for 5'2" Reese) would fit right in on some sunny, Italian-waiter-strewn patio. If you think gold sandals are too dressy for day, a neutral version, or some '40s-style peep-toes, would knock this look down a bit.

## Creative

**KIRSTEN DUNST remixes ingenue:** Creative layering can get garish, but this combo is sweetly, quietly cunning. Kirsten slips a delicate tunic that might look too "little girl" alone over a casual three-quarter-sleeve tee. Demure yet cool.

*Thanks, Mom*

Selma's "dress" is actually one of her mother's old skirts.

*Basket Clutch*

A natural-fiber bag plays up the look's earthiness—and contrasts nicely with slick shoes.

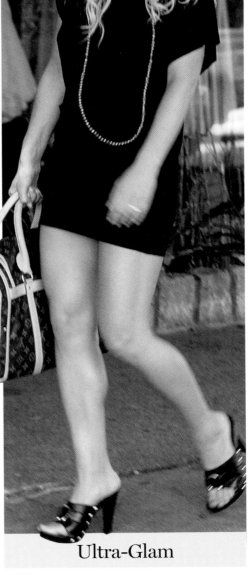

## All-American Sexy

**SELMA BLAIR in prairie chic:** Selma makes a comfy petticoat brunch-worthy with a massive warrior belt, transparent slides, and a ring that adds a welcome bolt of blue to all those earth tones. If you're not sure you could remain upright under her belt's crushing weight, anything dark and low-slung would do.

### Ultra-Glam

**JESSICA SIMPSON does "movie star":** Even in restrained daylight mode, Jessica compulsively wows in a plain black minidress, dramatized with a loop of beads and accessorized with a gigantic Louis Vuitton dog-tote.

# daytime date

The goal: an outfit that won't make *either* of you uncomfortable, even if he takes you **pumpkin picking on a whim.**

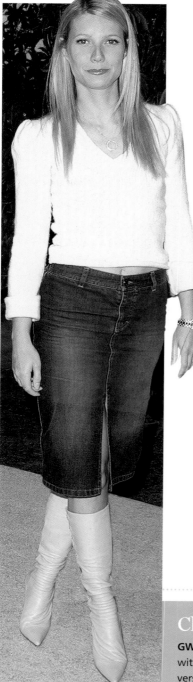

**How many of you have shown up** for a Saturday afternoon date and, ten minutes later, realized that your carefully labored-over outfit is not only itchy—but ill-suited for that spontaneously romantic walk down abandoned railway tracks? "Your date wants to go on a date with you, not your outfit," says Lynn Harris, relationship expert and author of *Breakup Girl to the Rescue!* Some bizarre and uncomfortable **Christina Aguilera**–style getup can bother him as much as it does you. "If you wear something distractingly flashy," says Harris, "it's like you're wearing stilts. He'll spend the afternoon staring at your stilts instead of listening to you."

What else you'll regret: skimpy clothes you'll freeze in, lawn-piercing heels, a clutch purse (think shoulder bag), anything motion-constricting, any top that requires you to sit at a rigid 93-degree angle so that your breasts won't tumble out. What looks right:

✳ **A LITTLE SEXINESS (NOT A LOT):** "If you're showing off your legs, cover up the rest," says celebrity stylist Tamara Rappa. "With sexy shoes, tear them down by wearing straight-leg pants, not a mini." (In stylist speak, "Tear them down" equals "balance them out.")

✳ **LOW-MAINTENANCE PIECES:** "Avoid anything that involves a lot of fiddling," says Harris, "like a floppy collar that has to be constantly adjusted so that it sits just perfectly inside your cute blazer's lapels."

✳ **DAY-APPROPRIATE FABRICS:** Cotton, knits, denim, wool. "If it's a miniskirt," says Rappa, "it better not be stretch satin." If you do wear a more sumptuous fabric like silk, tear it down (see how that works?) by pairing it with a more humble material.

## Classic

**GWYNETH PALTROW relaxes refinement:** No one wants to hang out in the park with some finicky *lady*. Gwyneth loosens up the pencil-skirt by choosing a denim version (with a slit for mobility), but keeps things girly with a puff-sleeved sweater.

"A date outfit should never say, 'I spent four days thinking about this outfit,' even if you did. You always want to look carelessly marvelous, like Daisy Buchanan in *The Great Gatsby*."

**–RELATIONSHIP EXPERT LYNN HARRIS**

## Creative

**MILLA JOVOVICH plays with prep:** A hacked-off mini, beatnik tights, and a cropped jacket hipsterize an Ivy League sweater. "With a miniskirt," says celebrity stylist Danna Weiss, "you run the risk of looking slutty if you wear something equally tiny on top. I'd also go for a cute dolman-sleeved sweater or a little hoodie sweatshirt."

### *Fringe Element*

The miniskirt's frayed hem nicely unsettles the conservative sweater.

### *Flat Boots*

Chic...and more practical than heels if you're dating an ardent *walker*.

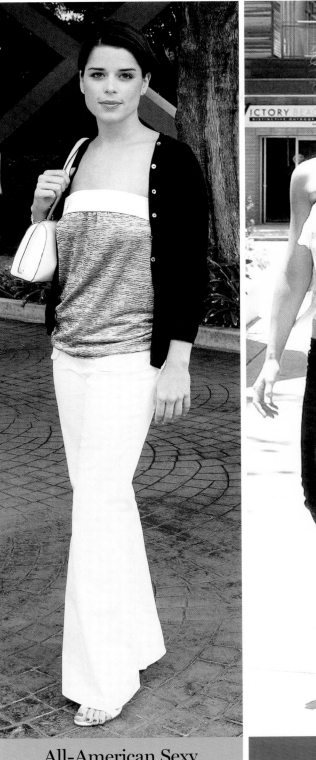

**All-American Sexy**

**Ultra-Glam**

**NEVE CAMPBELL chills out:** This easy look show-cases two sound date strategies: 1) A shoulder-strap purse leaves hands free for coffee or holding hands. 2) A cardigan, cozy if it gets cool, can always be dramatically shed if you want to show more skin.

**KATE BECKINSALE dolls up:** It's not just the slinky capris. Or the megaplatform shoes. Or even the nightclubby top. But when you put it all together with an updo and giant shades? Hello, ultra-glam! Some men might find Kate's look intimidating. The rest...won't.

# summer wedding

You want an outfit that's **dressy enough, yet not so glammy** that the bride starts glaring at you for distracting the groom.

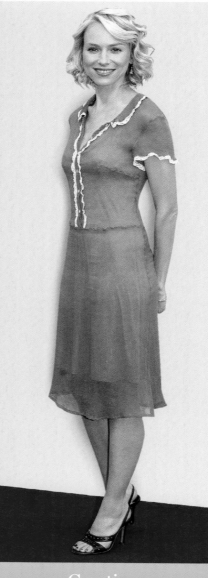

**Weddings come but 17 times a year** (or at least that's how it seems), and they always seem to hog the sunniest weekends. Naturally, you resent this. Not only must you dress up without challenging the bride's right to be the laciest and poofiest of all, you need an outfit that will look mysteriously breezy and picturesque in heat that could kill cattle. Star stylists advise:

**GO SLEEVELESS:** A floaty sleeveless dress with a drapey skirt is the safest bet if you want to be comfortable, appropriate, and sweat-stain-free, says stylist Tamara Rappa (who recently dressed pop star **Vanessa Carlton** for a wedding in a not-especially-safe red '20s flapper-style dress by Lela Rose). If you like your arms covered, layer on a delicate cardigan.

**LENGTH DETERMINES FABRIC:** "With a short dress, you can get away with more formal fabrics, like taffeta," says stylist Danna Weiss, "especially in lighter colors, like mint or beige. But if you're going full-length, stick to something airy—cotton or chiffon."

**DRESSES AREN'T REQUIRED BY LAW:** Though Rappa feels that suits have become an uncool wedding solution, tailored pants with a sleeveless top that's not too nightclubby would always work. "Or," she says, "you could do a simple top with an embellished skirt, maybe beaded chiffon, backed up with special accessories."

**DON'T EVEN THINK ABOUT IT:** Ugly crocheted shawls, Princess Diana hats, tights with sandals, lap dogs, black accessories, jean jackets, the orange satin bridesmaid dress you had to wear to some other wedding, your iPod.

## Classic

## Creative

**ERIKA CHRISTENSEN honors tradition:** With its sweetheart neckline, darted bodice, and full skirt, this floral dress evokes a '50s wedding guest (the sorority girl with whom the groom had a fling two years before.)

**NAOMI WATTS works '40s femininity:** To play up this dress's charming "run up on the sewing machine" quality, Naomi mixes in vintagey *brown* sandals instead of something more predictably, slickly "pretty."

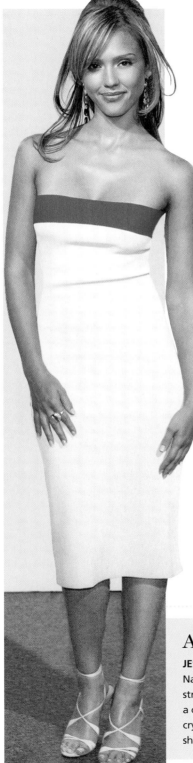

"Pantsuits look tired at a wedding now. We've moved so far from Helmut Lang minimalism toward girlier dressing that most suits feel stale, like something strictly office."

**—CELEBRITY STYLIST TAMARA RAPPA**

## Tie-on Fluff

A maribou-trimmed sash is a discreet amount of glamour. A boa is not.

## Walking Lessons Not Included

A dress this long is especially dramatic... when you trip on it.

## All-American Sexy

**JESSICA ALBA goes tubing:** This sexy Narciso Rodriguez dress—a tube top stretched into a cylinder of svelteness—has a cheerleader-fresh color scheme that's crying out for a green lawn. (In darker shades, it might seem *too* sexy.)

## Ultra-Glam

**ELLE MACPHERSON, looking 14 feet tall:** The ultra-glam woman habitually overshadows others, but even she has to respect the bride. Full-length dresses can be a bit much for a daytime wedding, but the soft femininity of Elle's ethereal halter gown makes it forgivable.

# Born Yesterday

Four classic celebrity daytime looks reinterpreted for the here and now

## Audrey Hepburn, 1954

Her suburban tomboy look moves into the city with more streamlined tailoring and posher textures.

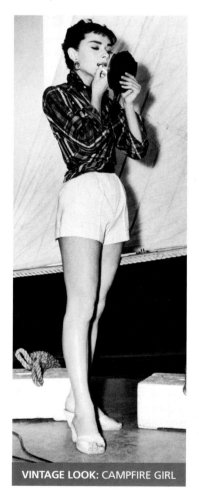

**VINTAGE LOOK:** CAMPFIRE GIRL

## MODERN TAKE: URBAN PLAYGIRL

**Modernize Audrey's togs** with a sleek tie-top specially cut to be less bulky than a knotted shirt, and low-slung shorts (in sophisticated tapestry cotton, not khaki).

*Hammered Gold Hoops*
More chic than classic tube-loops GIVENCHY

*Red Bag of Courage*
If your outfit's neutral, hit color with a bag. TOCCA

*Style-Conscious Wedgies*
Perforated pattern and peep-toe design—a step above pedestrian espadrilles C. RONSON

# Sophia Loren, 1955

A casual '50s dress gets booted up to superchic with more refined accessories

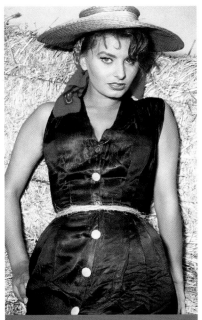

**VINTAGE LOOK: SHIRTDRESS SEXPOT**

## MODERN TAKE:
## SHIRTDRESS CHIC

Worn in the '50s by housewives, career girls, and the occasional sultry farm girl handy with rope, the shirtdress is most modern in black, particularly when paired with matching boots for a monochromatic head-to-toe silhouette.

*Head Scarf*
For extra star-quality
ADRIENNE VITTADINI

*Hobo Bag*
Relaxed but still dapper in black
DOONEY & BURKE

*What Tall Boots You Have*
The goal: no visible skin between boots and hem
COACH

## Twiggy, 1971

In the '70s, the manly suit wore the girl—all oversized slouchiness and vast lapels. Today, tough meets tender halfway.

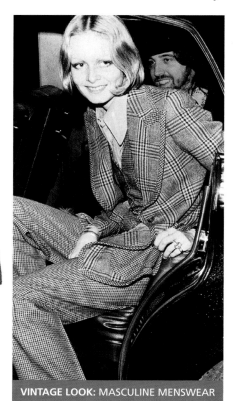

**VINTAGE LOOK:** MASCULINE MENSWEAR

### MODERN TAKE: FEMININE MENSWEAR

**What to keep:** The famously waifish model's mismatched tweeds. **What to lose:** Her blazer's sloppy proportions. A shorter, more fitted, ladylike jacket looks more modern, especially when dressed up with a gender blur of girly-tough accessories.

*Girly Brooch*
For a glint of feminine charm
RJ GRAZIANO

*Flashy Satchel*
Gold grommets glitz up
a heavy-duty bag. KOOBA

*Sexy Python Pumps*
More lithe than chunky boots,
but just as assertive
LUISA BECCARIA

### Neo-Charm Bracelet
A clean, millennial take on a clinking classic
H HILFIGER

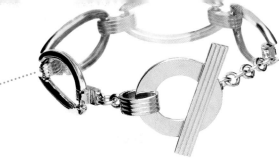

# Jacqueline Kennedy, 1962
Jackie's buttoned-up, white-gloved, White-House style comes undone in the Palm Beach sun.

### Huge Sunglasses
It's awfully sunny on the yacht. OLIVER PEOPLES

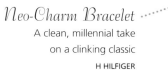

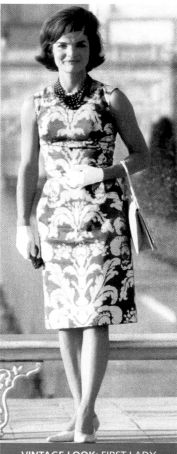

**VINTAGE LOOK:** FIRST LADY

### Big White Bag
Impractically white for that "the servants will clean it" look. BANANA REPUBLIC

### Jackie's Favorite Sandals
Modernized in silver
JACK ROGERS

## MODERN TAKE: PREPPIE GLAM

No one dresses quite *this* ladylike anymore, but that doesn't mean you can't channel Jackie's thoroughbred spirit. Update her stiff brocade sheath look with a preppie sundress (quirky enough that you won't seem cookie-cutter), and add accessories that say, "I'm rich…but, of course, you already know that."

**For full fashion credits, see page 221.**

# "JESSICA HAS REALIZED SHE DOESN'T NEED ALL THE BELLS AND WHISTLES."

—STYLIST RACHEL ZOE ROSENZWEIG ON JESSICA SIMPSON'S STYLE

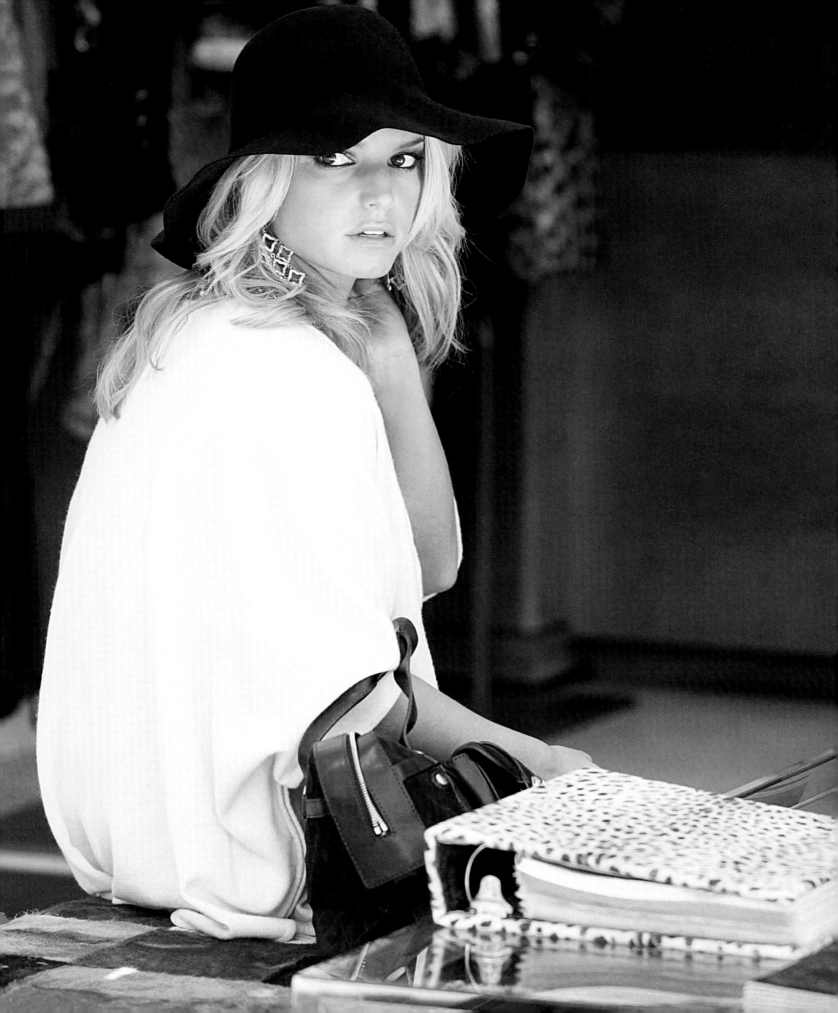

# chapter 8

# NIGHT OUT

We're not talking about a trip to happy hour. Or those post-work affairs that force you to transform yourself from worker bee to party girl in a bathroom stall. No, the focus here is on that special night out, the sort that inspires you to stick vague, exclamatory Post-Its on your computer: "Cocktail party! Clothes!?" It could be a friend's sit-down dinner party. A major date. Or a pivotal nightclub outing for which the style strategy can be summed up as "must look extra-hot to make ex-boyfriend jealous and regretful—ha!" Celebrities, especially free-spirited ones like **Drew Barrymore** and **Cameron Diaz**, go out more often than the ancient nomads did. And fortunately for those of us seeking style inspiration, celebrities (unlike nomads) never repeat an outfit.

"My boyfriend is out of town."

–DREW BARRYMORE, HERE WITH PARTNER-IN-CRIME, CAMERON DIAZ

# important date

**If he's made serious reservations** at a serious restaurant, it's time to break out of the standard jeans-and-cute-top formula.

**You know the formula:** Sexy jeans plus one of those flirty, droopy, wispy tops—as monotonously "different" as snowflakes. "I don't see the cute-top solution going away anytime soon," says celebrity stylist Danna Weiss, who's worked with **Molly Sims** and **Kim Cattrall**. "It's comfortable, it's easy, it's safe, and it's brainless." Maybe too brainless, says Jill Swid, **Uma Thurman**'s stylist, who thinks the cuteness epidemic has left a lot of women with fashion tunnel vision: "Everything's about the top now. It's a bore." While it's doubtful your guy has noted the tedium of cute tops just yet, why not shake it up? Our advice:

✳ **UNVEIL YOUR LEGS:** Remember legs, those things that give jeans shape? Though they lack decorative detail, in the eyes of many men, they are considerably "cuter" than any top.

✳ **GAMBLE ON GLAMOUR:** If he's gone out on a limb by planning a big date, take your own risk and wear an undeniably dressy dress.

✳ **EXPLOIT SENSUOUS TEXTURES:** If you're just not a dress person, stick with pants (even jeans), but really dress them up with a velvet jacket, for example, or a vintage angora sweater. As a seduction tool, texture can trump skimpiness, says relationship expert Lynn Harris: "In my experience, it's less about how much skin you expose, than how touchable you are."

*Gem-free*
Selma wears this LBD properly— with minimal jewelry.

*Drop Waist*
A half-belt gives the dress a subtle, retro, '20s quality.

*Hello, Toe*
Delicate bare shoes offset this dress's strength; closed-toe pumps would look too heavy.

## Classic

**SELMA BLAIR LBDs it:** For preppie sophistication, a Little Black Dress as elegant yet unassuming as this Calvin Klein version would look right at home in that restaurant you didn't even know he could afford.

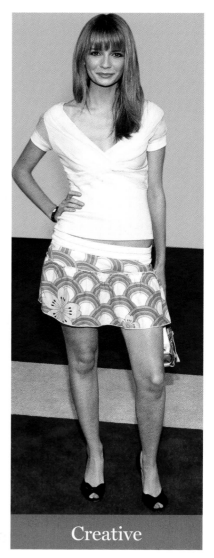

## Creative

**MISCHA BARTON keeps it pretty:** A fashionista mini and a gold Hogan bag—plus shoes in punky black— might be too much *fashion* for some guys, but Mischa lowers the intimidation factor with a simple chiffon top. Unless you're dating a man who knows who Dries Van Noten is, don't go too haute.

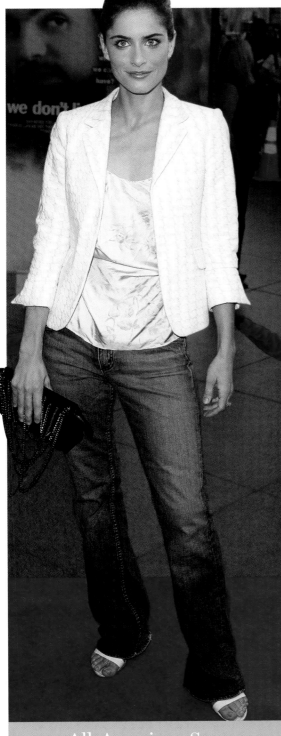

**All-American Sexy**

**AMANDA PEET takes denim further:** Amanda ups the sophistication of a routine cute top with a beautifully textured, cropped jacket. Nothing routine about that gem-spangled clutch, either.

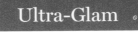

**Ultra-Glam**

**LINDSAY LOHAN does retro sex-kitten:** Gutsy color, elegant cut. Vintage-glam draping hugs Lindsay's cleavage (maybe you noticed) in a Valentino dress that seems designed to temporarily stun all men.

> "Denim is so mainstream now that women get very complacent. Sometimes you've got to have the guts to wear a dress."
>
> —JENNIFER RADE, **ANGELINA JOLIE'S STYLIST**

**STYLIST TIP:** If baring skin, don't forget the subtle erogenous zones: shoulders, clavicles, and the nape of the neck.

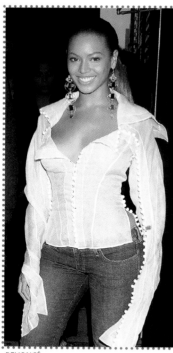

BEYONCÉ
too *octopus*

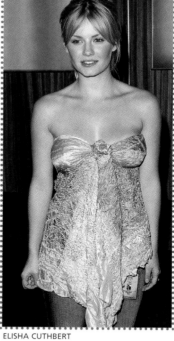

TARA REID
too *hobo*

ELISHA CUTHBERT
too *crumpled*

MISCHA BARTON
too *ticklish*

# the cute top hall of shame

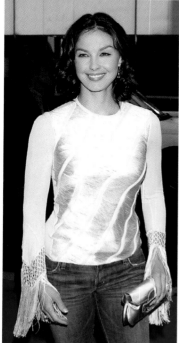

ASHLEY JUDD
too *figure-skater*

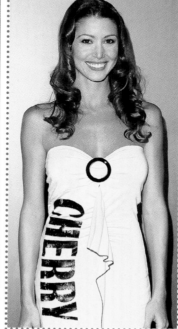

SHANNON ELIZABETH
too *chatty*

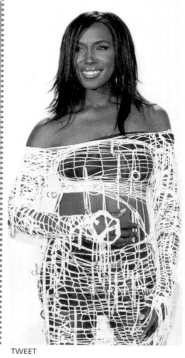

TWEET
too *strung-out*

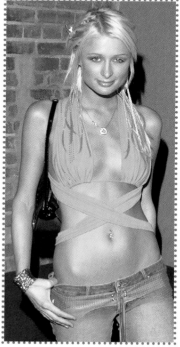

PARIS HILTON
too *modest*

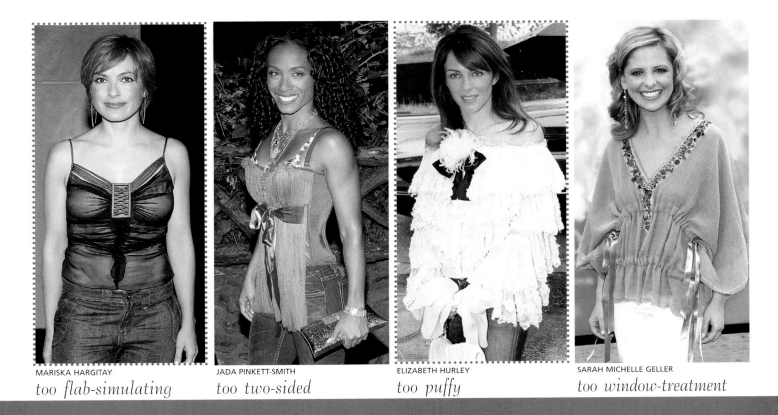

MARISKA HARGITAY
*too flab-simulating*

JADA PINKETT-SMITH
*too two-sided*

ELIZABETH HURLEY
*too puffy*

SARAH MICHELLE GELLER
*too window-treatment*

A so-called "cute top" and jeans. This combo has become America's standard date outfit, but beware: In a desperate quest for cuteness, **some tops try way too hard.**

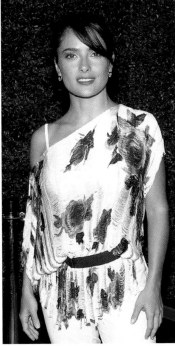

SALMA HAYEK
*too wilted*

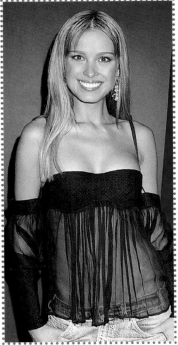

PETRA NEMCOVA
*too sleeves-sold-separately*

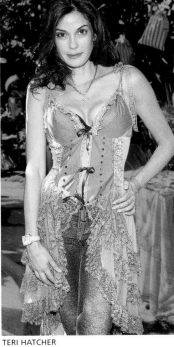

TERI HATCHER
*too wenchy*

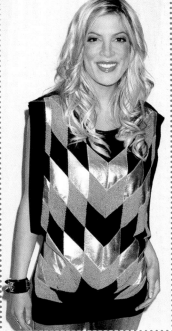

TORI SPELLING
*too bedspread*

# dinner party

How much to dress up, or down, when a friend (or enemy) is asking for RSVPs? **Best advice: Hedge your bets.**

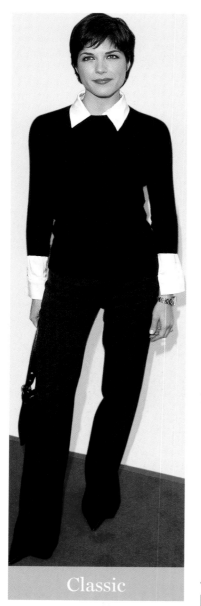

**Classic**

**SELMA BLAIR studies contrast:** Selma plays with proportion— a shorter sweater sleeve over a dangling silk cuff—to modernize a black-and-white look.

**"Having people over for dinner"** can mean so many things. If, as the day approaches, you've been getting breathless, squeaky calls from the hostess ("Help! What's fennel!?") chances are she's going all out and you need to make a fashion effort. (Now that private dinner parties have become an It event for stars like **Gwyneth Paltrow**, you're in good company.) "It's disrespectful if you show up looking sloppy, or hauling a giant tote overflowing with work," says celebrity stylist Tamara Rappa, who's dressed **Scarlett Johansson** and **Samaire Armstrong**. "When the point is to sit back and enjoy someone's effort, that's discounting her effort and the specialness of being *invited*."

If you really know the hostess, it's easier to get the dressiness level right. But what happens if you arrive at an acquaintance's home in your metallic capelet, and everyone else is wearing yoga pants and feeding infants apricot goo? Not such a tragedy: The beauty of pieces like capelets and beaded cardigans is that they're removable. If in doubt, dress in layers and subtract as required. "I usually tell people to take an extra pair of earrings," adds Danna Weiss. "If you get there and realize you overdid it with the huge, dangly chandeliers, just change into the studs."

*Swingy Charm*
Vintagey tassel pendants echo the shape of Kate's top.

*Extra Chill*
Note that Kate has unhemmed her jeans.

**Creative**

**KATE HUDSON has it both ways:** There's something grand about the Art Nouveau–inspired Chloe top that Kate's draped over denim. On the other hand, it's just a top and jeans, right? Not like she dressed up.

> "Trends are like fast food—it's easy to overindulge and overstyle yourself. A simple statement is always more elegant."
>
> **–MARY ALICE STEPHENSON, LIV TYLER'S STYLIST**

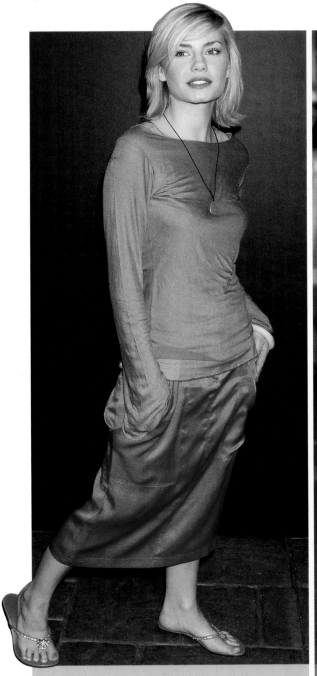

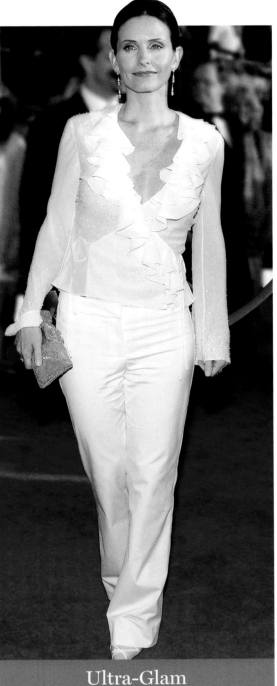

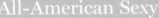

## All-American Sexy

**ELISHA CUTHBERT pushes the laidback limit:** Elegantly easygoing or too casual for a dinner party? Silky textures and the jeweled delicacy of Elisha's thongs make this a fairly safe bet—especially in summer.

## Ultra-Glam

**COURTENEY COX in stealth glitz:** How do glamour girls hedge their bets? They show up in a seemingly low-key Christian Dior top with crystal beading that begins to sparkle madly once the candles are lit.

# decoding the dress code

A guide to those wee invitation footnotes that supposedly tell you what to wear.

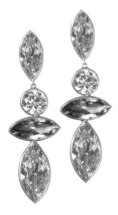

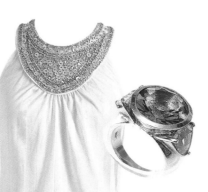

*"dressy casual"*

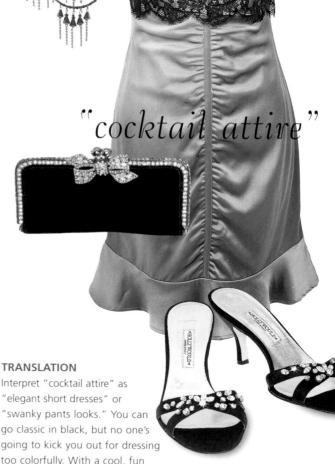

*"cocktail attire"*

### TRANSLATION

"Dressy casual" basically means "make an effort." No jeans, no shorts, no velour sweat suits. Wear the sort of clothes you find comfortable, but in brighter colors or more sensual fabrics (a shimmery tank, versus a plain cotton one).

### WHAT WE'D WEAR

A straightforward look with **Cameron Diaz**-ish twists: wool Theory pants with an unstuffy top (distinguished by a beaded crescent neckline). Plus: a pair of flirty ice-blue satin shoes, and pretty, but not wimpy, jewelry.

### TRANSLATION

Interpret "cocktail attire" as "elegant short dresses" or "swanky pants looks." You can go classic in black, but no one's going to kick you out for dressing too colorfully. With a cool, fun event, there's room for **Kate Hudson** sexiness, but if you foresee corporate types blathering on about real estate, think **Renée Zellweger**, and leave early.

### WHAT WE'D WEAR

We'd likely hedge our bets in a **Lucy Liu**-ish BCBG dress like this, sexy but ladylike, with accessories that pick up on its glitzy femininity.

# nightclub

There comes a time in every woman's life when **she wants to dance her butt off**, while radiating nuclear levels of sex appeal.

**You're going dancing.** Or maybe you're going to be "cramming into booths," that other popular nightclub activity. For single women especially, this is a rare opportunity to explore the dark art of Recklessly Foxy Style. Some tips on getting "hot" right:

✳ TWO WORDS: "Pushup bra," says Tamara Rappa concisely. If weekends were made for Michelob, dance floors were made for pushup bras.

✳ WEAR PLATFORM HEELS: "They're still sexy, but they give you more support than stilettos," says Rappa. "And whatever you do, don't wear those weird, small-heeled shoes. They make everyone look frumpy and middle-aged. Even flats are better."

✳ A LITTLE SKIN GOES A LONG WAY: "There's a lot of competition out there," says Danna Weiss, "but showing everything is not the way to compete. You need to work a little mystery." Not all of Weiss's celebrity clients have heeded this advice; she remembers trying to convince one (who shall remain nameless) to pair her favorite tiny top with a long, romantic skirt. "Unfortunately, she insisted on wearing it out with short shorts. It was tragic."

✳ JEANS AREN'T THE ONLY ANSWER: "A lot of women are sensitive about their thighs," says stylist Mary Alice Stephenson, who works with **Liv Tyler**. "In that case, it's about making a statement away from them. Keep it simple, *simple* on the bottom—a dark A-line skirt—then focus on a great pair of dangly earrings, or a necklace and cleavage." Pushup bra, anyone?

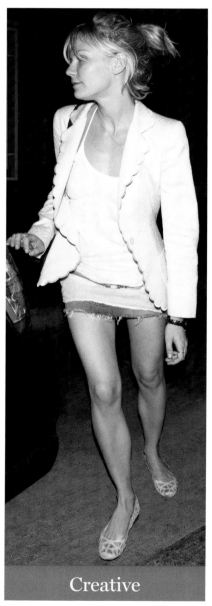

## Classic

**NATALIE PORTMAN as retro '30s fox:** Combining "ladylike" and "hot" is a Natalie specialty. You might argue that her glamour-puss '30s bob makes that top seem almost *too* elegant to co-exist with frayed jeans. But...why are you arguing with Natalie?

## Creative

**KIRSTEN DUNST keeps it loose:** Casual layers, twistily accessorized with a skinny disco belt and perforated flats. In a sweltering club, Kirsten could always lose the blazer (even though it has such cute scallop-edging).

> "Showing skin is not about shock value anymore—we've seen pretty much everything we can see. Now it's about intrigue."
>
> —CELEBRITY STYLIST DANNA WEISS

### Cap Sleeves
A ladylike look that Reese Witherspoon loves, too.

### Laced Up
A surprisingly "modest" neckline makes the top's sheerness more unexpected.

## Ultra-Glam

**CHARLIZE THERON underachieves:** Showing off your underwear can look cheap, but Charlize avoids trashiness by veiling her bra with a vintage-glam top that's both see-through and demure. Unlike Paris Hilton, who always goes too far, she's set her bling level on "low."

### Bootcut Jeans
Slightly flared, not too boxy, dependably sexy

## All-American Sexy

**AMY SMART rethinks cleavage:** This simple, plunging halter dress is both more—and less— risqué than your average skimpy top. Its "plainness" lets the complexity of Amy's sandals (and earrings) shine on nicely.

# cocktail party

When you're invited to a bona fide cocktail do, allow yourself some **bona fide glamour,** and don't worry about being overdressed.

**If you want an excuse** to really dress up, it's hard to beat a real cocktail party. (Not to be confused with a BYOB bash, or the 6 P.M. "corporate wine reception," for which only hateful, wrinkled work clothes are appropriate.) Most cocktail parties have a retro quality that makes them seem like they're taking place a long time ago in a galaxy far, far away, where denim doesn't exist yet. It's like everyone gets to play dress-up together—with none of that "why are *you* so dolled up?" paranoia. Accordingly, women sometimes go the retro style route in a little black dress like the one **Elizabeth Taylor** wears in *Butterfield 8*. Or even the sort of '20s flapper look that **Mischa Barton** has almost trademarked. And here it's important to listen to the experts: "When you're doing any retro thing," says Tamara Rappa, "don't wear the entire decade head to toe, or you'll look like you're going to a costume party." With a '20s beaded fringe dress, for example, don't overdo it by adding strands of necklaces *and* marcelled hair. Hats tend to cross the line. Danna Weiss agrees: "The risk of taking retro too far is that people might actually think they've seen a ghost." And fear isn't all that festive.

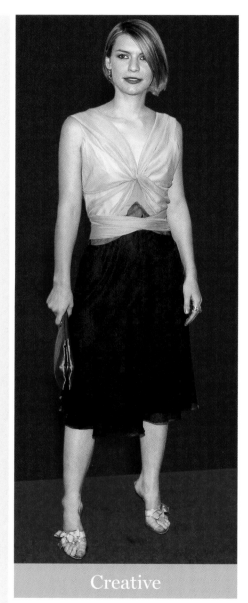

### Classic

**KATIE HOLMES plays by the rules:** A silvery top and black fluted silk skirt is a cocktail formula that's worked for decades. Katie plays out this traditional look from head to toe—with tidy hair and elegant slingback shoes. Her one rebellion: That chic chunky watch.

### Creative

**CLAIRE DANES works with color:** With its gorgeous mix of greens, this Prada dress is the sort of unique find that triggers jealous "where'd you get it?!" buzz at any party. When it came to accessories, Claire could have wimped out with neutrals, but chose unpredictable pinks, instead.

> "I'm completely behind the idea of women dressing up and looking as good as they can."
>
> –ELIZABETH HURLEY

## Tricky Toga

This Grecian-inspired gathered tunic looks great on Cameron, but that's a whole lotta fabric: If you're not so lean, look for a dress with a more defined waist.

## Statement Ring

Very Cameron: chipped nail-polish combined with a giant turquoise ring

## All-American Sexy

**CAMERON DIAZ ties one on:** This string-tied tunic is loose enough to wrestle in, but still dressy enough for any party, especially when accessorized with silver.

## Chain Metal

Sandals with a subtle gladiator vibe underline the dress's Grecian spirit.

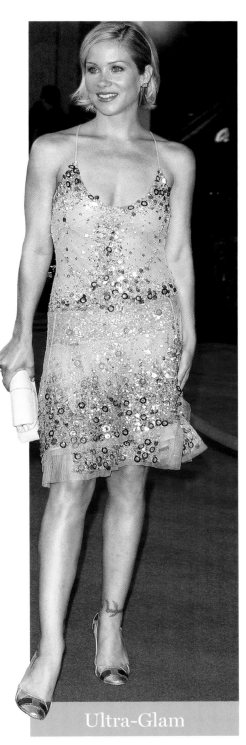

## Ultra-Glam

**CHRISTINA APPLEGATE shines complexly:** If you're a known glamour girl, everyone will be counting on you to really rise to the occasion. This chiffon dress by Blumarine, festooned with a seemingly endless variety of sequins, should keep the crowd happy.

# Pair Up for the Night

It's more modern if your accessories don't match, but they should still work together to personalize your look. Four duos that reflect the style—and designer allegiances—of four unique stars.

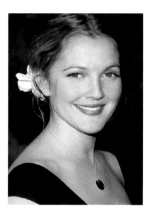

## DREW BARRYMORE
### *bohemian chic*

**Her go-to designer: STELLA McCARTNEY**

Vegan Drew, who's long supported McCartney's "cruelty-free" fashion, doesn't wear a lot of leather. These cow-conscious vinyl pumps—teamed with a turqoise-trimmed Oscar de la Renta bag—express Drew's haute-hippie style *and* her politics.

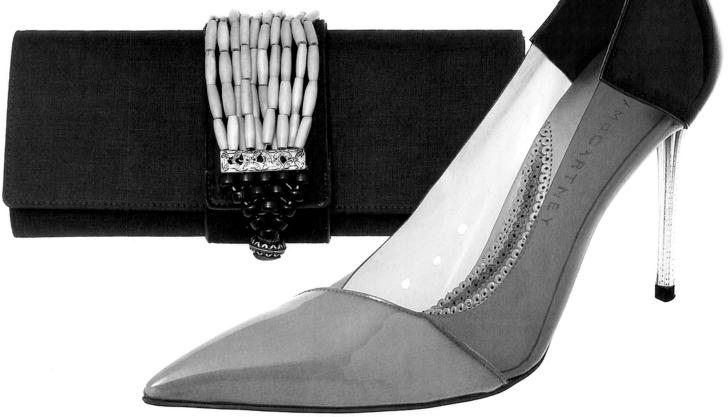

# REESE WITHERSPOON
## *ladylike preppie*

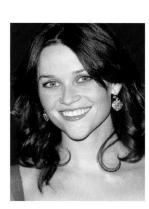

**Her go-to designer:** MICHAEL KORS

Reese has worn a lot of hot pink in her movies, but her personal style is more subdued. Kors' croc bag (paired with murkier blue H Hilfiger peep-toes) is suitably quiet, but not boring.

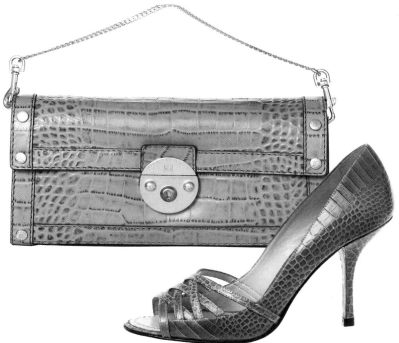

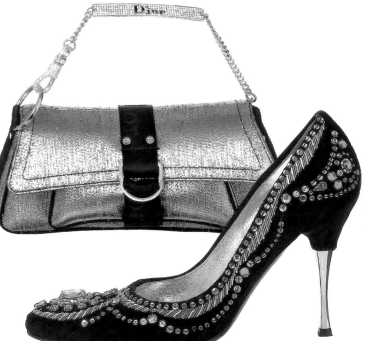

# EVE
## *fierce*

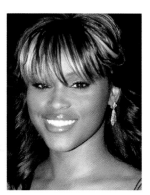

**Her go-to designer:** CHRISTIAN DIOR

Though Eve often carries bags from her own Fetish by Eve line, Dior's flash also catches her eye. A characteristically unshy combo: Dior's metallic evening bag and jeweled Sergio Rossi pumps.

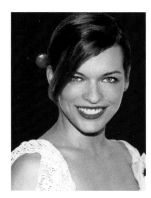

# MILLA JOVOVICH
## *eclectic glam*

**Her go-to designer:** CHRISTIAN LOUBOUTIN

It's only natural that Milla, whose own clothing line Jovovich-Hawk, is influenced by the '40s, would dig the classic sexiness of Louboutin. A typically creative Milla mix: his pink satin heels with a vintagey python bag by Clara Kasavina.

"IT WILL
BE NICE
TO LOOK
BACK
AT PHOTOS
AND SAY,
'AT LEAST
I'M WEARING
CLOTHES.'"

—MANDY MOORE ON WHY SHE DOESN'T GO OUT IN SKIMPY THINGS

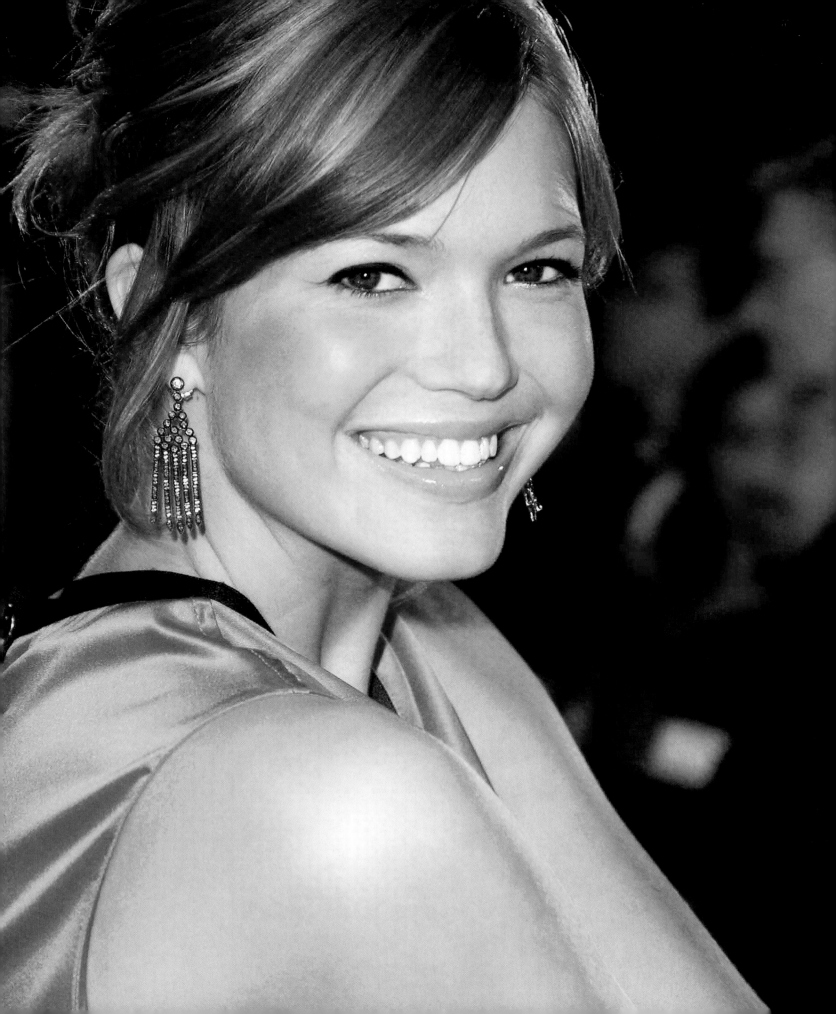

# chapter 9

# BIG EVENT

OK, think fast: For reasons too complex to explore here, you've just been invited to attend the Oscars. What do you wear? Good question. Naturally, you don't want to overshadow **Gwyneth Paltrow** too badly. Or make **Gwen Stefani** so jealous she'll challenge you to a tense sing-off. But you still want to earn your share of admiring "who's that?" stares and briefly incapacitate **Jude Law**, who'll likely want to sit on your lap at some point in the evening. Clearly, you need to find a dress that's dead-on right for you. That should be the goal for *any* major event in a woman's life: Prom, for starters. A lavish wedding, a New Year's gala, that benefit you have to attend next month because your boss "strongly suggests it." So think fast: What will you wear, this time for real?

"My mom made me a dress exactly like Grace Kelly's in *Rear Window*."

—GWEN STEFANI ON HER HIGH SCHOOL PROM

# prom

**Puffy princess gowns will always have their fans, but if you want to go more modern (or actually dance), abdicate the throne.**

*Sweet Rocks*
Big, pompous jewelry would be the ruin of this innocent look.

**Prom is the Oscars for teens.** Stretch Hummers. Parents doing their dorky best to impersonate paparazzi. And tons of pressure to get the dress right, which, especially for girls who view prom as a dress rehearsal for their weddings, often means princessy ballgowns. Sara Rogers, a trend expert with the Mall of America in Bloomington, Minnesota, doesn't expect the great tradition of stuffing crinolined girls into limos to die anytime soon. But, she says, more sophisticated teens want to look like **Mischa Barton** or **Kate Hudson**, not Scarlett O'Hara: "After Kate wore a yellow dress in *How To Lose a Guy in 10 Days*, we had girls everywhere asking for that precise color." They likely found it, thanks to labels like ABS by Allen Schwartz, which sells clones of the stars' gowns for less than $400. "The celebrity influence on prom looks in the past few years has been huge," says Schwartz, who names **Natalie Portman** and **Scarlett Johannson** as inspirations. Our advice:

✳ **WALK AWAY FROM THE GOWN:** Consider the sort of ultra-dressy shorter looks that Scarlett and **Mandy Moore** wear. For the price of a ball gown, you might be able to score a designer find on sale.

✳ **DON'T FORGET YOUR BODY:** You may like a celebrity's look, but that doesn't mean it's right for you. Mischa's slinky red gown over there might look skanky on someone really busty.

✳ **KEEP IT LIGHT:** Or bright. Black may increase the odds that you'll look dignified in photos years from now, but c'mon! It's prom.

## Classic
**EVAN RACHEL WOOD in retro ballerina:** A ballerina-length formal—like Evan's Oscar de la Renta dress with its lush flutter of chiffon leaves—is a cooler take on traditional than a blah, tulle floor-length ball gown.

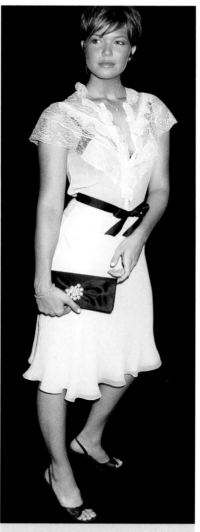

## Creative

**MANDY MOORE flirts with lace:** A shorter retro '40s dress like this Oscar de la Renta number redefines the modern prom look, especially if you edge up its ladylike laciness with a slightly boyish haircut and a glimpse of pretty black bra.

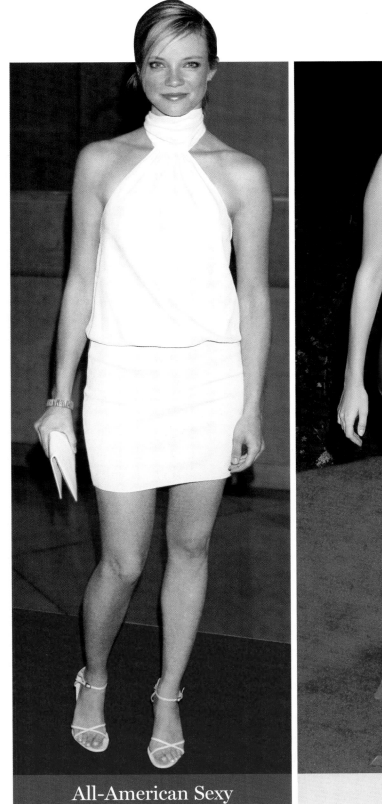

## All-American Sexy

## Ultra-Glam

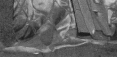

**AMY SMART goes for freedom:** It takes guts to rebel in a Giorgio Armani halter dress this simple (even if it's "formal" white), but some girls would rather dance and hang out with the funny guys than bob around the room in a 9-foot-wide blimp gown.

**MISCHA BARTON loosens up full-length:** Ideal for cutting-edge high school divas with no interest in looking "sweet." With its slash cutaways, this Roberto Cavalli slip dress would scandalize all the chaperones, even if it weren't flaming red.

# formal wedding

**The challenge here:** To balance a certain respect for the occasion with an impulse to wear something absolutely, inappropriately fabulous.

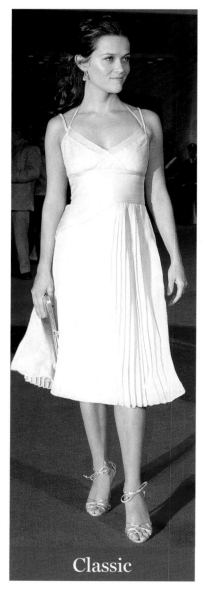

**Classic**

**REESE WITHERSPOON says grace:** Cool in a good-girl way, this subtly intricate chiffon Carolina Herrera dress is both respectable and (especially around the neckline) sexily sheer. Minimal makeup helps.

A formal wedding has a higher degree of fashion difficulty, but the upside is you really get to dress up. Even so, says stylist Erin Hirsh, who works with **Eve**, it's better to subdue the glamour. A sequined wrap, for instance, is fine, she says, if the sequins are a neutral color: "You have to follow an unwritten rule of respect. The focus isn't on you. And you don't want to be the girl who's making everybody whisper, 'She looks ridiculous.'" Subdued, maybe, stodgy, no, says celebrity stylist Tamara Rappa, who recently attended a Turkish society wedding at New York City's swank Rainbow Room: "You never want flashy, but it's more modern to go fashion-forward. And short." (In case you're wondering, she wore a black, beaded, knee-length Badgley Mischka dress with a pink satin Kate Spade bag.) Other considerations:

✳ **WEDDINGS CAN LAST FOREVER:** Especially if the groom gets drunk and makes the band play "Come On, Eileen" so repeatedly that your Pavlovian response to dance to that song finally breaks down. So don't wear anything uncomfortable, stifling, or worrisomely revealing.

✳ **DON'T WEAR A SHAWL TIED BEHIND YOU:** "Terrible look," says Rappa. "Sandra Bullock did it in *Two Weeks Notice*, even though her character was this chic woman who normally wore Prada." If you wear a shawl, capelet, or stole, choose one that fastens with a ribbon or button.

✳ **USE ACCESSORIES TO MODULATE YOUR LOOK:** "If your dress is fairly fabulous, cool it with simple accessories," says Hirsh. And vice-versa.

## Creative

**SARAH JESSICA PARKER remixes the past:** She blends textures (downy, gauzy, shiny) and vintage influences into a pretty look that exemplifies modern wedding-guest style. The winner of the most original shawl-alternative prize: Her puff-sleeved jacket.

*Get a Bead on It* SJP's bag, encrusted with multicolored crystals, adds just enough glitz.

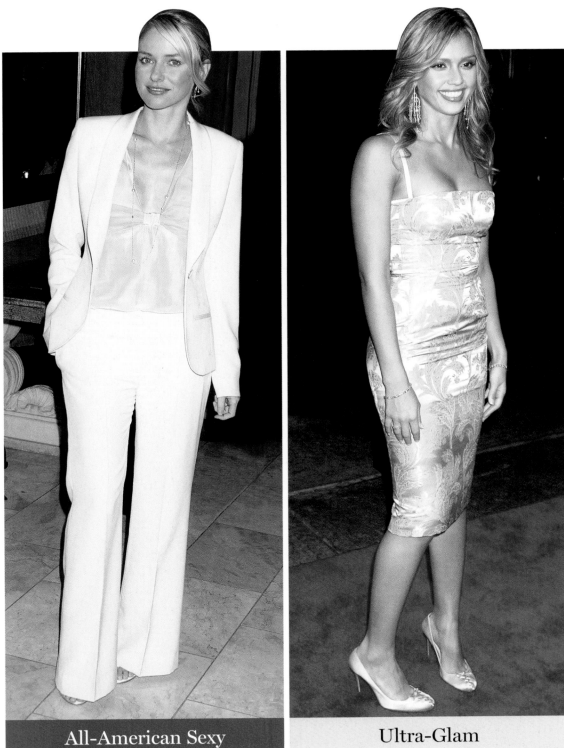

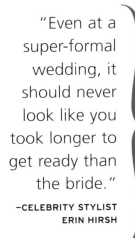

## All-American Sexy

## Ultra-Glam

**NAOMI WATTS arouses trousers:** A suit can work for a formal wedding if it looks as if it's never been anywhere near a stapler. Naomi achieves sensual elegance with tuxedo-style shawl lapels and a camisole so flesh-colored it's more topless than top.

**JESSICA ALBA in corseted brocade:** This Dolce & Gabbana sheath is totally sexpot, but those Christian Louboutin stilettos have enough of a matchy bridesmaid vibe to make the look wedding-friendly—especially for boring guests who need something to gossip about.

# black-tie affair

The actual black tie is his problem. All you have to do is find the **most beautiful dress in the universe.** (Hey, no pressure.)

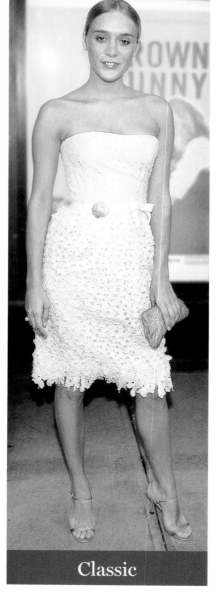

**At a black-tie gala, you're free to really work it,"** says celebrity stylist Erin Hirsh, who helps mastermind **Eve**'s funk-glamour look. "And I think most women want that opportunity." That means buying a truly remarkable dress or a full-length gown, a process that can trigger a whole range of emotions—delight, insecurity, competitiveness—as well as a fair amount of self-delusion, says stylist Tamara Rappa (who recently accepted the challenge of dressing the 4'11" L'il Kim for a gala event): "A lot of women are, like, ooh, it's finally my chance to wear a fuchsia strapless dress. But strapless is not that flattering on most people, especially if it hasn't been fitted. So they end up pulling up their dress the whole night, and having a rotten time." Make sure that's not you:

✳ **KEEP IT SIMPLE:** "A black-tie event is not the time to try a trend," says Rappa. "You don't do the crazy color, you don't do the offbeat." Choose a fairly classic gown, she advises, and wear it with delicate, elegant jewelry. "Nothing too costumey and plasticy."

✳ **REMEMBER YOUR BODY:** "When women are buying a formal gown, they sometimes forget all the years they've spent learning how to dress their figures," says Hirsh. "The key is to pick a dress that shows off your favorite part. Try spaghetti straps if you like your upper body. Or a slit, if you think your legs are hot." (For more on gown figure flattery, see page 142.)

✳ **TRY ON EVEN THE LOSERS:** A gown that looks sad on the hanger can turn out to be the answer. Trust us on this one: Zipping on a multitude of gowns is the best way to learn what works for you.

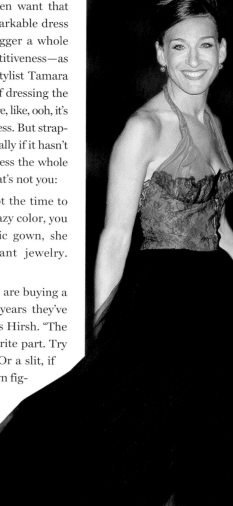

## Classic

**CHLOE SEVIGNY in petal white:** Though cocktail-length, this Oscar de la Renta eyelet dress—seemingly made of apple-blossoms—is easily special enough for black-tie. Precise ballerina hair ups the formality factor.

## Creative

**SARAH JESSICA PARKER laces up:** A collectible '50s formal is a unique way to sidestep the gown predictability issue. In this vintage Howard Greer dress, Sarah Jessica reminds us of the hot Latina chick in *Grease* who steals John Travolta from Olivia during the dance contest. Except not so dastardly. And much more sophisticated.

> "The rules say you can wear pants to a black-tie gala. But, to me, those women just never look chic."
>
> **—CELEBRITY STYLIST TAMARA RAPPA**

*Loose Hair*
With a dress this sexy, don't go the stiff-updo route.

*Eye-Catching Detail*
If you're going to work a silver accent here, be willing to be thoroughly admired.

## All-American Sexy

**JENNIFER ANISTON** buckles under: A modern take on formal, this vintage Valentino gown has been widely copied for obvious reasons—it's simple, it's hot, and that hypnotically positioned buckle, reminiscent of overalls, toughens up its sexiness. (A bow would have had a completely different effect.)

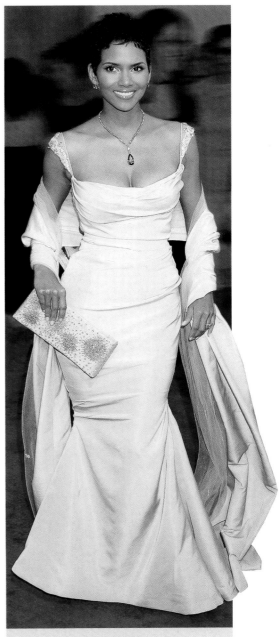

## Ultra-Glam

**HALLE BERRY does diva:** If you aspire to full-throttle Oscar-level glamour, this off-the-shoulder Halle gown—with a matching wrap that serves no purpose except to trail behind you inconveniently, but regally—would certainly fit the bill.

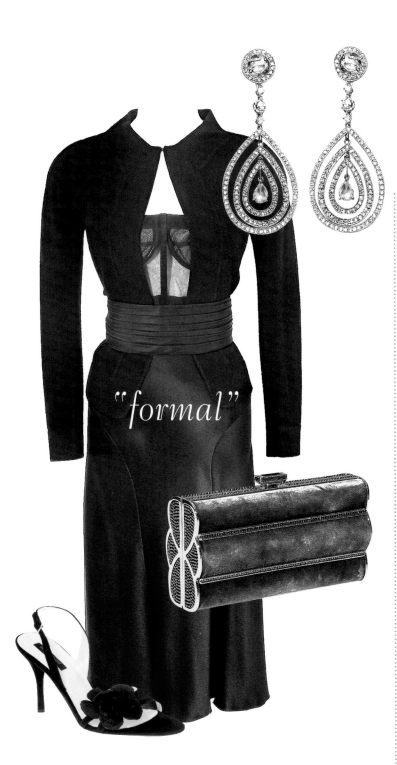

## "formal"

### TRANSLATION

Serious glamour. A sophisticated dress, either short or full-length, or ultra-refined separates. If you're going to go short, look for a dress that reflects some or all of these key terms: special, serious, unforgettable, actually fits.

### WHAT WE'D WEAR

We'd probably rebel, and bypass a dress for the sort of sexy skirt look you'd see on **Naomi Watts** or **Jennifer Connelly**, like this Monique Lhuillier ensemble with a sheer bustier. Plus: a Deco-style clutch and some blinding rocks.

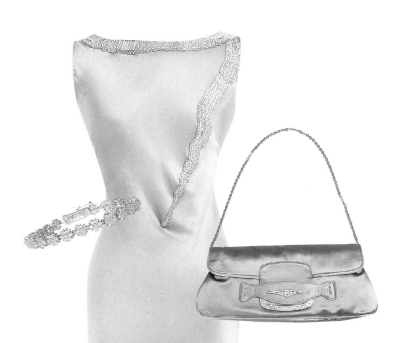

## "black tie"

### TRANSLATION

Essentially the same as "Formal," though with a stronger suggestion that you wear a long gown. While a short dress or evening separates are still acceptable, if the invitation says "White Tie," you are absolutely required to wear a formal full-length dress, or fear the consequences.

### WHAT WE'D WEAR

Something classic with a retro twist, like this '30s-inspired Alberta Ferretti gown, with its serpentine ribbon of rhinestones (very **Nicole Kidman**). And we'd be careful to respect its simplicity with quietly sumptuous accessories. **For full fashion credits, see page 221.**

# Gownology 101

A guide to Hollywood's top 12 styles, from traditional ballgowns to retro-'70s streamlined halters—one for every figure and personality.

## 1. Bustier

### Sarah Jessica Parker
**AT THE 2003 EMMY AWARDS, IN CHANEL COUTURE**

With built-in bustiers so structured they defy gravity, these dramatic gowns usually work best on chestier women who can really fill them out. In Sarah Jessica's case, strategic neckline poofiness simulates the va-voom effect, and softens it. (She's wisely pulled her hair back so it doesn't compete for poofiness dominance.) Though she's said this dress was the "easiest thing I've ever had to wear," eyewitnesses report that she spent a fair bit of time tugging it up, a potential problem with any bustier gown.

✳ **BEST FOR:** Hourglass figures; those with killer-instinct flair

✳ **NOT GREAT FOR:** Small-breasted women; nervous recluses

# 2. Beaded

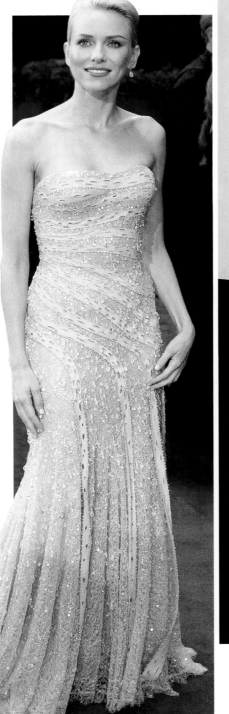

## Naomi Watts
### AT THE 2004 ACADEMY AWARDS, IN ATELIER VERSACE

The upside of beaded gowns is their wow factor. The downside: They're not exactly feather-light (up to 20 lbs.), and can snag on everything from cutlery to your escort's piercings. In 1930s Hollywood, costumers would spend up to seven weeks systematically beading an entire gown. Although Naomi has said she chose this Swarovski crystal-encrusted version for its "old-school glamour," its beading has a modern, more loosely crafted look.

✳ **BEST FOR:** Those who are willing to pay for quality work

✳ **NOT GREAT FOR:** Comfort addicts; younger women (head-to-toe beading can look old— look for some beaded detailing, instead)

## Kristen Davis
### AT A 2004 LONDON EVENT, IN ALEXANDER MCQUEEN

Trapeze gowns make a strong, A-line statement. Their slightly shapelier cousin, the empire-waisted gown (fitted through the bust), is more common, but both designs offer regal, demure silhouettes that lend themselves to sweeping entrances, and a simplicity that can make petite women look taller.

✳ **BEST FOR:** Shorter or pear-shaped figures; pregnant women; minimalists

✳ **NOT GREAT FOR:** Hourglass figures; sexpot show-offs

# 3. Trapeze

# 4. Retro-Inspired

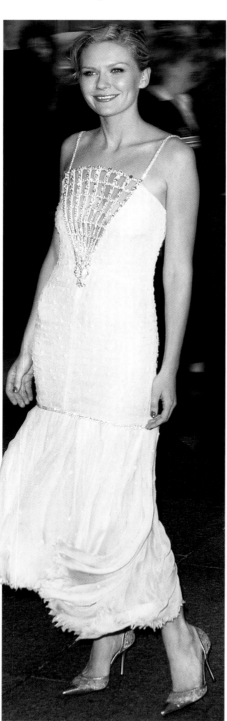

## Kirsten Dunst
AT A 2004 LONDON
PREMIERE, IN CHANEL
COUTURE

With the exception of certain determinedly modern Japanese designs, almost every gown is *somehow* retro. Hollywood's golden age from the '30s to the '50s remains the biggest style influence. Less tapped-out decades include the '20s, '60s, '70s, and (you better be brave) '80s. The advantage of going retro: Originality gets you noticed. There's nothing Miss America–generic about Kirsten's gown, with its '20s-style drop waist and Art Deco–influenced rhinestone neckline (perfect, incidentally, for smaller-breasted women).

✳ **BEST FOR:** Risktakers; anyone who's into fashion history

✳ **NOT GREAT FOR:** Those who like to stay in their comfort zone; Miss America

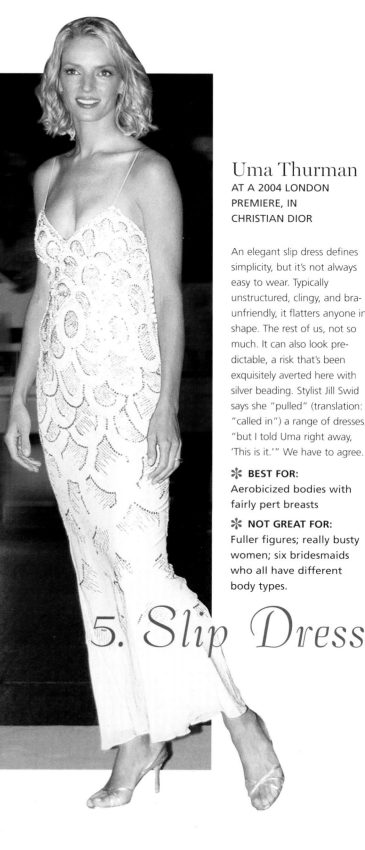

## Uma Thurman
AT A 2004 LONDON
PREMIERE, IN
CHRISTIAN DIOR

An elegant slip dress defines simplicity, but it's not always easy to wear. Typically unstructured, clingy, and bra-unfriendly, it flatters anyone in shape. The rest of us, not so much. It can also look predictable, a risk that's been exquisitely averted here with silver beading. Stylist Jill Swid says she "pulled" (translation: "called in") a range of dresses, "but I told Uma right away, 'This is it.'" We have to agree.

✳ **BEST FOR:** Aerobicized bodies with fairly pert breasts

✳ **NOT GREAT FOR:** Fuller figures; really busty women; six bridesmaids who all have different body types.

## 5. Slip Dress

# 6. Asymmetrical

## Jennifer Garner

AT THE 2004 ACADEMY AWARDS, IN VINTAGE VALENTINO

Asymmetrical necklines, great for women with toned upper bodies, guarantee you'll look distinctive. "Jen likes her neck and shoulder area," says celebrity stylist Rachel Zoe Rosenzweig, who chose this one-shouldered chiffon dress, originally designed in 1973, to showcase them both. "She just loved it, and her confidence came through on the carpet." (It's an example of a dress that had no "hanger appeal," as Rosenzweig puts it. "When Jen first saw it folded over the hanger, she didn't even want to try it on. It looked like nothing, some orange sheet. I'm not kidding.")

✳ **BEST FOR:** Small-to-medium busts; women who want a clean, modern look

✳ **NOT GREAT FOR:** Bigger busts

"Couture never looks uptight on Halle—it looks sexy. She has the curves and the right attitude to warm up intimidating clothes."
**—DESIGNER MARK BADGLEY OF BADGLEY MISCHKA**

# 7. Ball Gown

## Halle Berry
**AT THE 2000 EMMY AWARDS, IN VALENTINO**

With its structured, waist-defining bodice and hip-concealing tent of a skirt, a ball gown can make many women look good, even majestic. The most traditional silhouette, it skews "bride," so avoid white, something Halle clearly considered. (Strapless versions like hers need to fit really well in the bodice; work closely with a seamstress. No one wants to see flab overflow, so if you're not that toned, consider a higher, less form-fitting neckline.)

✳ **BEST FOR:** Both thin and hourglass figures; pear-shaped figures; romantics

✳ **NOT GREAT FOR:** Shorter women (its width makes them look squat); anyone who wants to look more fashion-forward

## Julia Roberts
AT THE 2004 ACADEMY AWARDS, IN GIORGIO ARMANI

This much-copied dress—made especially for Julia—is all about vintage glamour. Seemingly improvised (notice how she appears to have been wrapped up, cinched, and broached just seconds ago?), the look dates back to the '30s, when couturiers designed gowns by draping fabric over a model and pinning it in place. It's sexy and decidedly grand, but all that material does add bulk.

❋ **BEST FOR:** Hourglass figures; anyone aspiring to high glamour

❋ **NOT GREAT FOR:** Fuller or pear-shaped figures

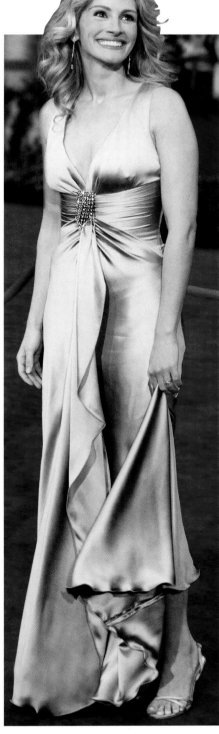

# 9. Halter

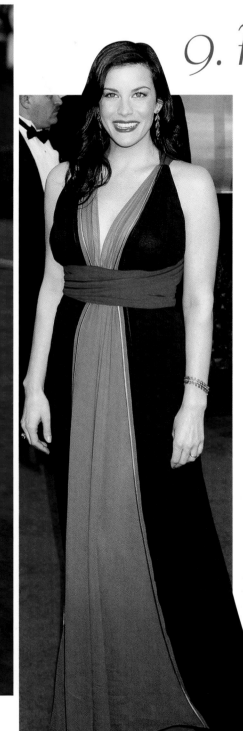

## Liv Tyler
AT THE 2004 SCREEN ACTORS GUILD AWARDS, IN MARC JACOBS

The halter design is bold, strong, and very American. Its vertical emphasis typically makes women look taller and thinner. This silk crepe georgette version—one of our favorite gowns ever—is a bit of a rebel, since that red horizontal waist-sash interrupts all the thinning verticality. But the primary goal here was clearly drama, and Liv completely pulls it off.

❋ **BEST FOR:** A range of figures (try it), including pear-shaped; those with narrow shoulders

❋ **NOT GREAT FOR:** Anyone who prefers a delicate, superfeminine look.

# 8. Goddess

# 10. Halter-Loop

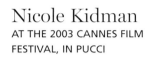

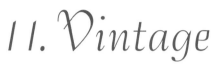

## 11. Vintage

### Nicole Kidman
AT THE 2003 CANNES FILM
FESTIVAL, IN PUCCI

A close relative to the classic
halter gown, this cut also does
amazing things for your shoulders, but it's less revealing—a
good choice if you don't have
much to reveal. There are endless
variations on the halter loop or
tie (in Nicole's case, a customized
jeweled choker by Bulgari worn
with matching cuffs). Go glitzy or
simple, depending on your taste.

✳ **BEST FOR:** Small-
breasted women

✳ **NOT GREAT FOR:** Bustier
women; anyone with saggy
shoulders

### Julia Roberts
AT THE 2004 SCREEN
ACTORS GUILD AWARDS,
IN VINTAGE VALENTINO

Among the most memorable
dresses in recorded human history, this circa-1982 gown (in black
velvet with white piping) demonstrates the value of going vintage. For those without personal
stylists, working the vintage angle
can require a certain zeal for
shopping or eBaying, and luck
(not to mention tailoring), but
the payoff is often worth it.

✳ **BEST FOR:** Adventuresses;
fashion hounds

✳ **NOT GREAT FOR:** The lazy

> "I hate stealing the show, but I'd worn a lot of black, covering-up things, and I thought... not this year."
>
> **–KATE WINSLET ON WEARING RED**

## Kate Winslet

**AT THE 2002 ACADEMY AWARDS, IN BEN DE LISI**

By definition, sheath gowns hug your body from the bust down to the thighs. They often involve an undercorset with built-in boning, so they're not exactly relaxing, but, if you don't mind taking a night off from breathing, few gowns are more classically stunning. (Flexible plastic boning is generally more comfortable than steel.) At the time, Kate said, "I wouldn't want to have to pee at this moment," but she did report that the comfort level was "actually pretty high."

✳ **BEST FOR:** Hourglass figures; thin women; shorter women

✳ **NOT GREAT FOR:** Pear-shaped figures; anyone who wants to nod off to sleep in her gown

# 12. Sheath

# PART FOUR

STRAT

Thinking Like A

Almost every star has a stylist—
or two—with assistants, and a Blackberry, and a
subtly controlled sense of panic. As you can imagine,
it's not easy to dress someone who's photographed
constantly from every angle. Especially when the star
has a tricky body, or a sudden craving for a gold lamé
beret. Or a baby on the way. We've all faced similar
fashion challenges (even if the closest we've come to
the paparazzi is Kevin the annoying cousin who *loves*
his new digital camera). And that's when insight into
celebrity stylists' strategies really comes in handy.

# Celebrity Stylist

# chapter 10

# ANY-FIGURE

Just a guess but, as you flip the pages of this book, is the following thought echoing through your head? "But I'm not built like some celebrity—how am *I* supposed to wear these clothes?!" Remember, even celebrities aren't built like celebrities. For every **Charlize Theron**, there are umpteen stars whose bodies fall short of the humbling Charlize ideal. **Cynthia Nixon** is as relatably hippy as your best friend. At 5'2", **Reese Witherspoon** is a stylish shrimp, while unbosomy **Debra Messing** has become a master of cleavage-simulating chic. **Oprah**, of course, has had every type of body. But lucky for the rest of us non-Charlizes, stars don't always ace their figure challenges, which allows us to learn from both their fashion hits and misses. (Note to Charlize: You might even want to take a look.)

"I'm not small and curvy—I don't meet the prerequisite for passive, sexy chicks."

—NICOLE KIDMAN, HERE WITH OPRAH WINFREY

# short

Say yes to long, lean shapes. Say no to anything that makes you look like a **souvenir doll from Austria.**

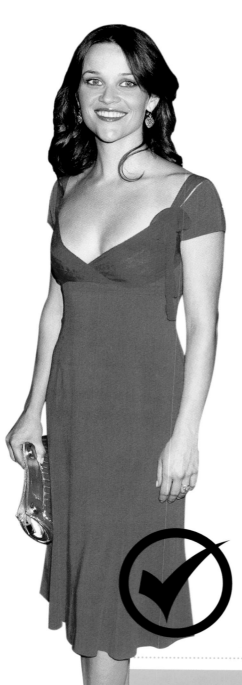

**Great things come in small packages,** but it helps if the packaging is streamlined. If you wrap yourself up in a giant fake-fur chubby jacket like the one that recently victimized 5'1" **Hilary Duff**, you'll look like a particularly squat panda. Not a hot look. Follow **Reese Witherspoon**'s lead, at left, and wear fitted, simple clothing that's scaled to your body. Then people won't think "short," or attempt to pet you. They'll just think "well-dressed."

GO FOR

❋ **Clean shapes:** You want clothes that adhere closely to your body's lines—sleek (but not tight) dresses, single-breasted jackets, flat-front pants.
❋ **Heels:** Wedge, kitten-heel, stiletto, anything except shoes with heavy ankle straps, which tend to shorten and thicken legs
❋ **Knee-length skirts:** A thigh-revealing slit helps.
❋ **Compact accessories:** Giant bags, belts, scarves, or jewelry can dwarf you.
❋ **Extra-long jeans:** Jack them up with heels so they graze the floor. Result: Another three inches of "leg."

DON'T BOTHER WITH

❋ **The "chop' effect:** Any outfit that sharply divides your top and bottom with color or a bulky waistband
❋ **Cuffed or cropped pants:** Rolled jeans included
❋ **Infantilizing details:** Ruffles and bows can make you look like a little girl, emphasis on "little."
❋ **Anything oversize or bulky:** Sloppy cargo pants, *Flashdance* sweaters, ponchos, puffy ski jackets, excessive **Olsen twin**-style layering

## Streamline your look

Clean silhouettes, like Reese's body-skimming Alberta Ferretti dress, help shorter women appear taller. Bonus: This dress's high empire waist creates the illusion that her legs begin near her ribs (don't think too hard about that).

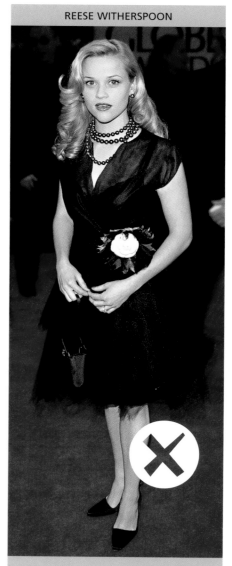

REESE WITHERSPOON

## Steer clear of crinolines

Avoid clothes that widen your look. See how this crinoline-inflated skirt thickens Reese into squatness? Other teensifying factors: the oversize pearls and flower, both out of proportion with her petite frame.

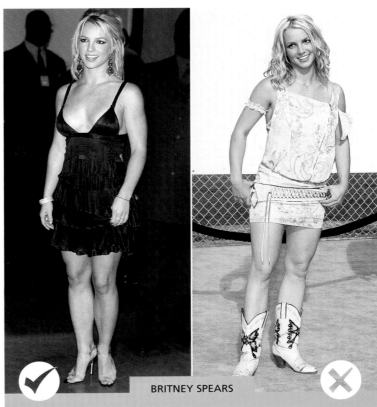

**JADA PINKETT-SMITH**

**THINK SOLID COLOR:** A column of cream makes 5'0" Jada seem statuesque.
**NOT TWO-TONE:** When color cuts her body in half, she seems to shrink.

**BRITNEY SPEARS**

**CHOOSE INVISIBLE SHOES:** Barely-there sandals lengthen 5'4" Britney's legs.
**NOT CLODHOPPERS:** Boots chop her stems into stubs, especially with a miniskirt.

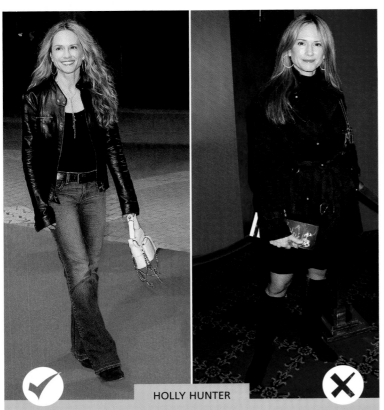

**HOLLY HUNTER**

**GO FOR FITTED:** Holly willows up in a lean-cut jacket scaled to her 5'2" body.
**NOT FLAPPY:** This bulky, double-breasted trench coat swamps (and shortens) her.

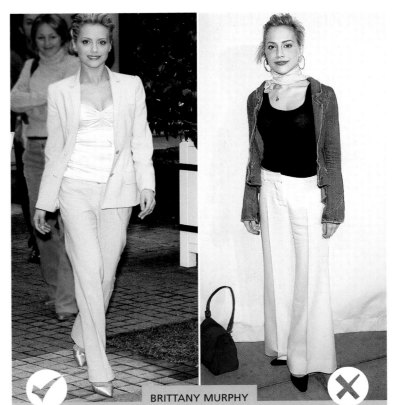

**BRITTANY MURPHY**

**WORK STRAIGHT PANTS:** In tailored trousers, 5'3" Brittany walks plausibly tall.
**NOT VAST BELL BOTTOMS:** Certain sailors might consider this look flattering.

# small bust

**If your cups runneth** on the small side, work the sleek, chic clothes other women can't wear.

**"I would never have surgery,"** none-too-busty **Jennifer Garner** once joked. "But it would be so much easier to get a boob job than to constantly have to find ways to pad out my cleavage." If you're small on top, focus less on the interminable quest for padding (even a Wonderbra has its limits), and more on choosing cuts that play to your strengths. Unlike those women who are weighed down with superboobs that distort their silhouettes, you can wear a lot of the high-end fashion that's designed for boyish models: jackets that need to hang just so, wispy summer dresses, chunky turtlenecks. Of course, not *everything* flatters you. (That'd be too easy.)

### GO FOR

❋ **Halter necklines:** An ideal cut to show off your shoulders (and back), instead of breasts.
❋ **Subtle revelations:** Unbutton a white shirt, or try the old fitted-blazer-with-nothing-underneath trick.
❋ **Girly details:** Test out tops and dresses with ruching, ruffles, or draping across the bust.

### DON'T BOTHER WITH

❋ **Structured bodices:** "Sexy" corset tops and dresses become counterproductive if you can't fill them.
❋ **Scoop necks:** They leave nothing to the imagination.
❋ **Clingy fabrics:** Unless you're working that strung-out, Estonian model vibe. But that's your business.

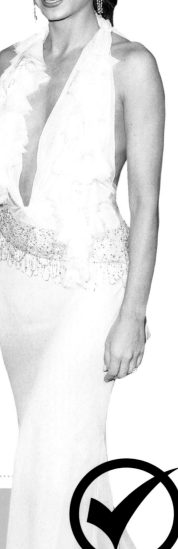

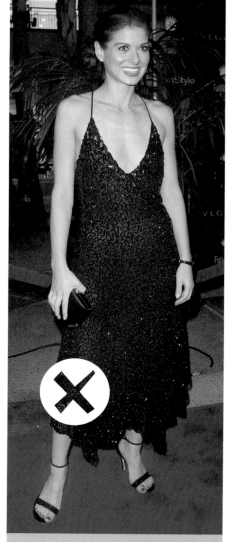

DEBRA MESSING

### Cut to the chase

Cleavage isn't everything: Debra shows off a tantalizing sliver of skin in a Vera Wang halter gown with a deep-V neckline (softened with strategic ruffles). This dress—a powerfully persuasive argument against getting implants—wouldn't sit correctly on a much bustier woman.

### Resist saggy slip dresses

Debra makes a rare misstep in a neckline that leaves her overexposed. This might have worked better if the dress had been cut much higher—then the focus would be on her dramatic collarbones (a classic Audrey Hepburn move).

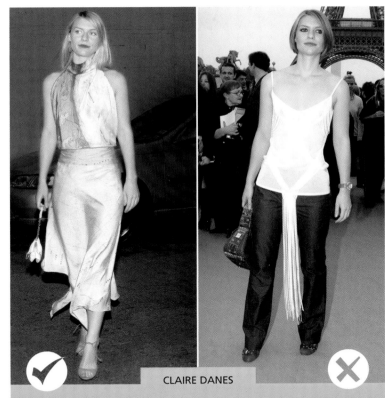

**CALISTA FLOCKHART**

**TRY A SHEATH:** Calista has the perfect figure for a classic tailored sheath dress.
**BUT SHUN TUBES:** Clingy tube-top things can look (and feel) deflating.

**CLAIRE DANES**

**WORK A HIGH HALTER:** Busty women just can't wear this sophisticated style.
**NOT A LOW-CUT TOP:** Sure, it's skimpy, but we think Claire looks sexier on the left.

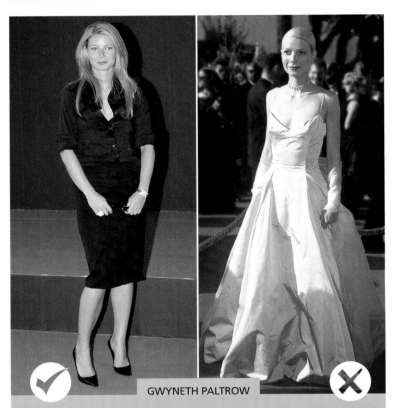

**GWYNETH PALTROW**

**COME UNDONE:** Small-busted women can unbutton any shirt tastefully.
**NOT UNFITTED:** Avoid structured bodices you're not equipped to fill out.

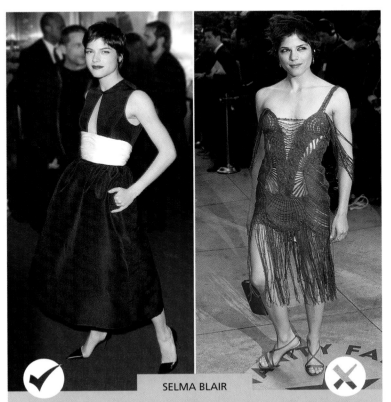

**SELMA BLAIR**

**SHOW SKIN STRATEGICALLY:** A surprising cutout sexes up Selma's formal dress.
**NOT COBWEBBISHLY:** Though clever, spiders know nothing about figure flattery.

# pear-shape

If you're hippy, soft draping and vertical lines are your friends. **Stovepipe jeans are not.**

**It's great that Beyoncé Knowles**, who's anything but model-thin, says empowering things like, "Women should embrace their curves. You don't have to be a size 4 to be beautiful!" But how exactly to proceed with all this curve hugging? Beyoncé loves taut pencil skirts that mold her superbooty into a **Sophia Loren** swell of sexiness, which works if you've got the chutzpah (and the waist) to pull it off, but is hardly the only option. If you prefer to embrace your curves more discreetly, you can still be a tasty pear.

## GO FOR
* **A-lines:** Softly flared skirts and dresses tend to downplay the swell of your hips.
* **Dark bottoms:** Ditto on that.
* **Boot-cut pants:** Avoid super low-rise styles; they should sit above the widest point of your hips.
* **Lower necklines:** Emphasize cleavage to balance yourself out. (A Wonderbra can be handy.)
* **Shoulder boosts:** Consider a jacket with modest shoulder padding to widen your top half.

## DON'T BOTHER WITH
* **Waist details:** They just attract attention.
* **Pleats or draping:** Anything that bulks up the hip area is generally not a great idea.
* **Tapered pants:** A.k.a. your nemesis.

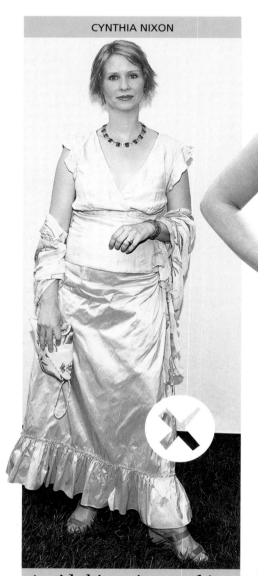

CYNTHIA NIXON

### Avoid shiny pioneer skirts

Three reasons to stay far away from metallic skirts: 1) They make everyone look bulkier; 2) They attract the eye ("Ooh, shiny!"); 3) Do you really want to hypnotize the public with your bulky, shiny hips? (Giant ruffles aren't such a hot idea, either.)

### Go with the flow

Cynthia looks hot in a soft chiffon, A-line Escada dress that sexily balances out her figure. Cleavage becomes the focus here, and a fluttery, uneven hemline (instead of one that cuts straight across the body) further de-emphasizes hips.

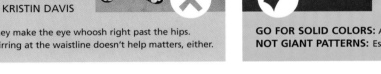

KRISTIN DAVIS

**PLAY UP VERTICAL LINES:** They make the eye whoosh right past the hips.
**NOT HORIZONTALS:** Bulky shirring at the waistline doesn't help matters, either.

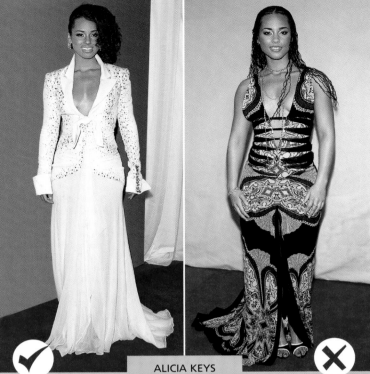

ALICIA KEYS

**GO FOR SOLID COLORS:** A relatively simple, ivory gown streamlines Alicia body.
**NOT GIANT PATTERNS:** Especially a print that fiendishly expands where you do.

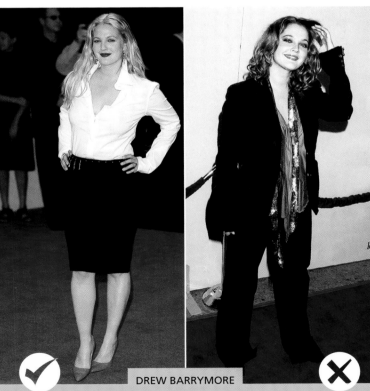

DREW BARRYMORE

**SHRINK HIPS IN DARK BOTTOMS:** A black pencil skirt shifts the focus up top.
**NOT SLOPPY TOPS:** Swath yourself in droopy fabric and *everything* looks bigger.

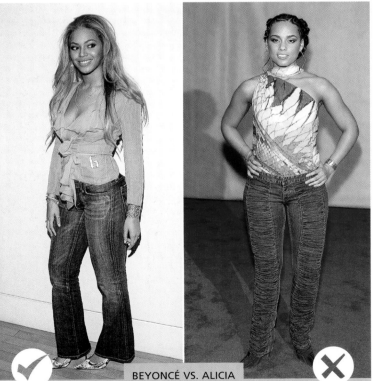

BEYONCÉ VS. ALICIA

**WEAR BOOT-CUT DENIM:** Beyoncé counteracts hippiness with a flared hem.
**NOT TAPERED JEANS:** Alicia, well, doesn't.

# big bust

An overflowing bra isn't necessarily a blessing. Choose the wrong cut, and you risk the **dreaded "bread loaf" effect.**

**When Pamela Anderson was in junior high,** some guy poured water down her shirt and yelled, "Now maybe they'll grow!" They eventually did, under a plastic surgeon's supervision, but Anderson (who's said that her favorite hobby is "upholstery") eventually came to regret her much-ogled, unwieldy implants. Major cleavage is a powerful asset, but it comes with a price: Hide it under conservative necklines and you can look lumpy; show it and people have a tendency to stare. If you're comfortable revealing at least some skin, however, it's not that hard to look tastefully sexy.

## GO FOR

✳ **Relatively open necklines:** You're not really built for the buttoned-up look. Anything V-neck is usually a good option for you (we're even talking T-shirts, here).
✳ **Fitted jackets:** For a less-exposed evening look.
✳ **Wrap dresses:** Useful for embracing your curves.

## DON'T BOTHER WITH

✳ **Bulky or shirred fabrics:** Padding you don't need.
✳ **Thick waistbands:** See Salma Hayek, right.
✳ **Shiny fabrics:** In certain kinds of light, they can literally give you headlights (and, for similar reasons, never wear gauzy dark materials over white bras).

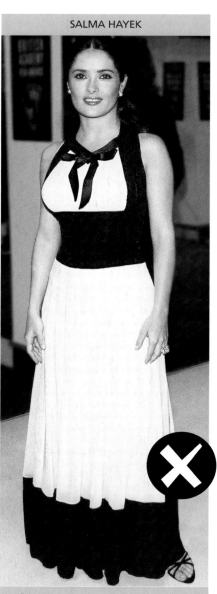

SALMA HAYEK

### Avoid mono-boob

In this unfortunate "peasant gown," Salma seems to have just one large rectangular breast, a condition known variously as "mono-boob" or "the bread loaf." To blame: An overly high neckline, plus a thick, contrasting waistband that turns her bosom into a shelf.

## Skin is not a four-letter word

When it's appropriate, choose a neckline that reveals enough skin to balance out your bust. A lot of women might find Salma's Narciso Rodriguez gown intimidatingly tight or *too* revealing (and not exactly bra-friendly). Find out what works for you.

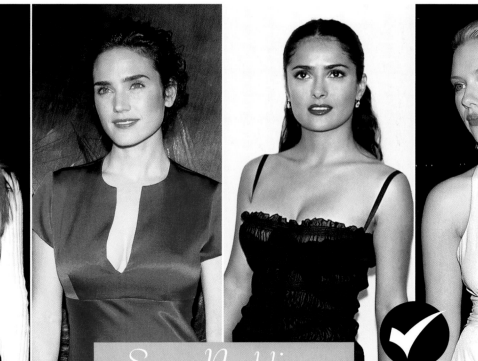

## Sexy Necklines

✓

**SCOOP NECK**
In classic white, JESSICA SIMPSON shows enough skin to balance things out.

**SLIT-FRONT**
JENNIFER CONNELLY finds a more modest alternative to a wide-open neckline.

**CORSET-STYLE**
Bust-embracing bodices like this were invented for women like SALMA HAYEK.

**PLUNGING HALTER**
The classic Marilyn Monroe solution, reinterpreted by SCARLETT JOHANSSON.

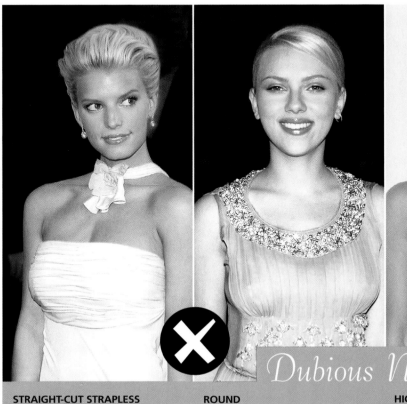

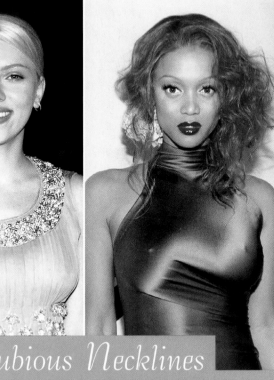

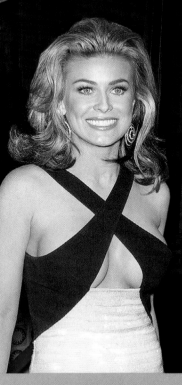

✗

## Dubious Necklines

**STRAIGHT-CUT STRAPLESS**
JESSICA's boob-tube style is hard to wear. Try a sweetheart neckline, instead.

**ROUND**
In this classic cut, SCARLETT JOHANSSON looks top-heavy and oddly matronly

**HIGH HALTER**
Not for the bodacious—on TYRA BANKS, shiny fabric magnifies the problem(s).

**SLING-SHOT UNDERCLEAVAGE**
This might be a sexy look, if CARMEN ELECTRA stood on her head.

# full-figure

**Not everyone was born to be stick thin.** But that doesn't mean you need to hide out in drab, unsexy clothes.

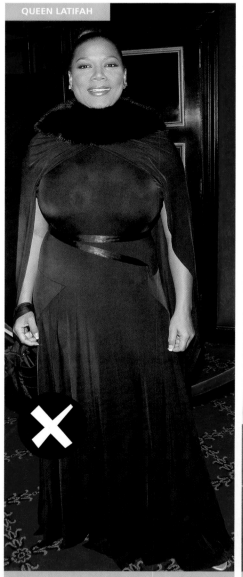

QUEEN LATIFAH

### Black isn't always slimming...

**Queen Latifah, before a 2003 breast reduction:** In this quasi-medieval look, she's so covered up, there's almost no visible skin (not even a neck) to offset her bust. When you're this swathed and layered, even in "flattering" black, you look anything but slim.

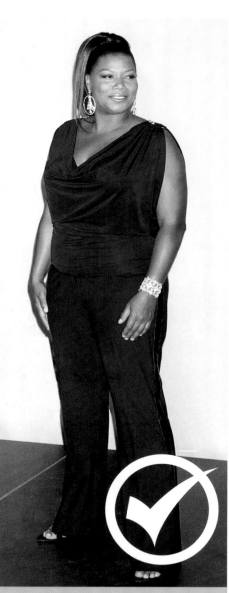

### ...but it can be, if done right

**After her reduction:** Looking much better in black, and not just because her chest is more streamlined. Now that she's showing some cleavage, her curves are working for her. (If you prefer not to show your upper arms, try a fluttery cap-sleeved top.)

**One of the key rules of style:** Dress the body you have right now. Don't think, "I'll just hold off buying anything new until I lose X number of pounds." It's always good to set a goal, even better to reach it—but why walk around in a less-than-flattering wardrobe until you do? Even if you're fine with your shape as it is, don't work against your figure with clothes that just don't fit. **Oprah Winfrey**, who's had her share of different bodies over the years, rarely wears anything that doesn't fit her perfectly, one reason she (almost) always looks great.

### GO FOR

✳ **Strategic fabrics:** Look for materials that aren't too clingy, especially if they're thin.
✳ **Wrap dresses:** Especially in darker colors
✳ **V-necks:** They can help elongate your neck.
✳ **Tailored clothing:** Pieces with defined waists can help give you an hourglass look.

### DON'T BOTHER WITH

✳ **Shiny fabrics:** They make everyone seem bigger, and not in that fun, larger-than-life way.
✳ **Shapeless pieces:** Ponchos, oversize tees, and tent dresses will leave you looking sexless.
✳ **Unnecessary bulk:** Pleats, ruffles, drawstring pants, too much layering, double-breasted jackets, trenchcoats, arctic-explorer fur

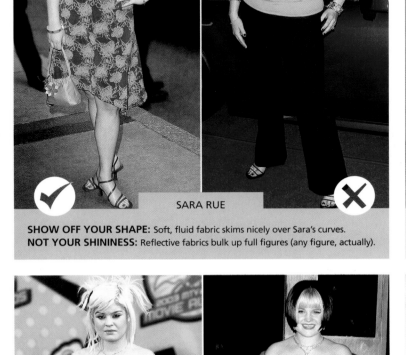

SARA RUE

**SHOW OFF YOUR SHAPE:** Soft, fluid fabric skims nicely over Sara's curves.
**NOT YOUR SHININESS:** Reflective fabrics bulk up full figures (any figure, actually).

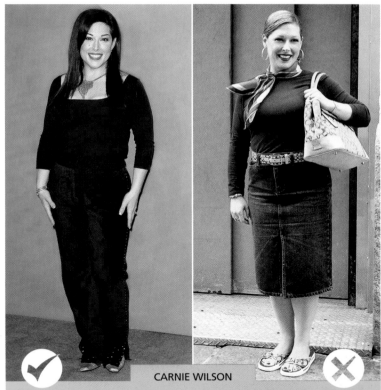

CARNIE WILSON

**WEAR STRONG ACCESSORIES:** Carnie can get away with a bold necklace like this.
**NOT ALL AT ONCE:** If she lost the scarf or belt (or both), she'd have a cleaner look.

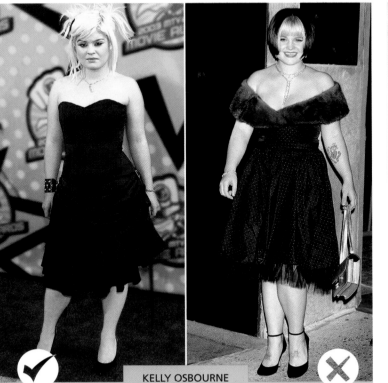

KELLY OSBOURNE

**THINK CORSET:** Kelly goes punky sexpot in a waist-creating little black dress.
**NOT FURBALL:** She invests unwisely in fur. (Even her hair has its own mink stole.)

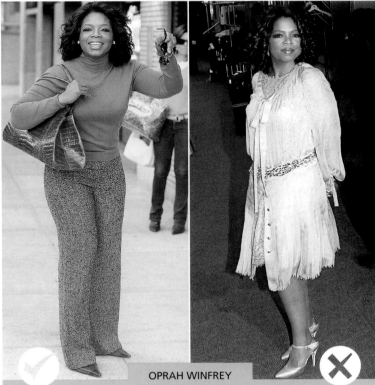

OPRAH WINFREY

**CHOOSE TAILORED LOOKS:** Strong color can rock if the clothes fit really well.
**NOT FLOUNCY MESSES:** Clearly, one of those "what was I thinking?" moments.

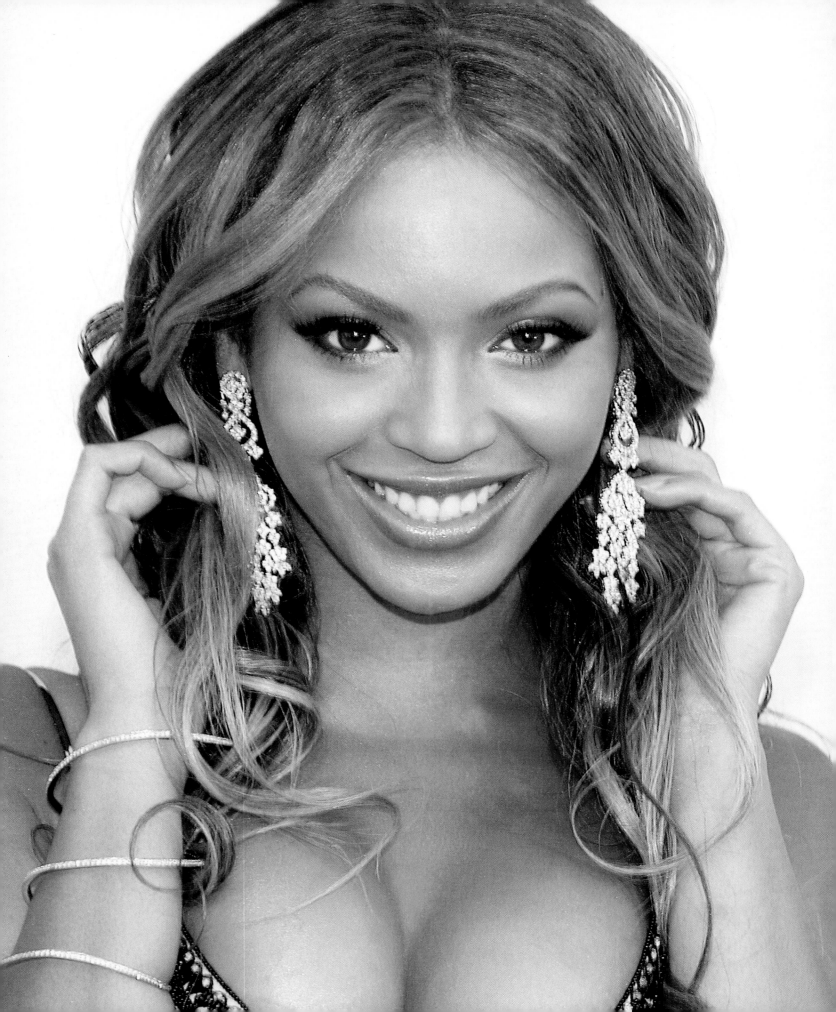

"RAIL-THIN MODELS MIGHT LOOK GOOD ON THE RUNWAY, BUT IT'S WOMEN WITH CURVES, AND A BUTT, WHO LOOK GOOD IN REAL LIFE."

—DESIGNER DONATELLA VERSACE ON BEYONCÉ

# chapter 11

# BUMP CHIC

Celebrities are at their most real when they're pregnant. Once the bump begins to show, they take a well-deserved break from being impossibly perfect. Their faces soften. They relinquish their hard-won abs. Stars who once leapt from limos in a blur of lanky legs are content to mosey along. In some ways, what changes the least is their style. Though the little black dress must become a sizable black dress, and tiny camisoles give way to industrial-strength bras, pregnant stars like **Gwyneth Paltrow** and **Kate Hudson** still want to look chic. They bare their bellies in Chanel harem tops, wriggle into knee-length sweater dresses, sling belts across their bumps, and if that all sounds impossibly stylish, don't worry. They also love their yoga pants, the roomier the better.

"I'm not giving up my high heels."

–A NEWLY PREGNANT KATE HUDSON (SHE EVENTUALLY DID), HERE WITH NAOMI WATTS

# everyday style

Even when their bumps are really bulging, the stars dress (more or less) the way they always did. And that's **triggered a maternity-wear revolution.**

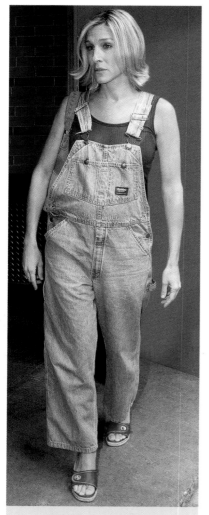

## '70s Comfort

**SARAH JESSICA PARKER** goes earth-mama in adjustable OshKosh overalls, but de-slobs the look with her inevitably cute shoes. "Overalls are a tough look for the average pregnant woman to pull off," says Lange. "Look how skinny Sarah Jessica is!"

During her 2004 pregnancy, Gwyneth Paltrow dressed with her signature sophistication—only bulgier. **Sarah Jessica Parker** did not disappear inside dorky tent dresses just because she was with child. "Celebs stay true to their style," says Skye Hoppus, co-owner of the hip Los Angeles maternity line, Childish, which custom-made Gwyneth's favorite pregnancy jeans, a low-rise vintage cut designed to sit under the belly. Hoppus (who's married to Blink-182 frontman Mark Hoppus) has found that most fashion-forward women want to hang onto their everyday cool through all three trimesters. "The conservative woman has always had options," she says. "But, until celebrities helped create a market, more daring women really didn't." When **Debra Messing** was spotted with a decidedly unmatronly Mickey Mouse halter-tee embracing her bump, women from Texas to Ohio tried to order that exact top, says Jennifer Noonan, owner of the L.A. maternity boutique NOM: "Sometimes, it was hard explaining that it was a customized vintage tee." NOM, which also dressed **Jennifer Aniston** for *Friends* during her character's pregnancy, eventually turned out more than 500 one-of-a-kind variations on this hot item. Gwyneth wore hers, belly prowing out from under its kitschy dragon motif, on the cover of *W*, the hautest of America's high-fashion magazines.

Even 10 years ago that would have been unthinkable. Maternity wear had traditionally been baggy and uncool, with no risk of visible navels or serious fashion cred. "Everything was oversize and babyish, with Peter Pan collars," says designer Liz Lange, who first pioneered chic maternity clothes in the mid-'90s. "The real change lately," she says, "is that, partly thanks to Hollywood, maternity clothing looks exactly like non-maternity clothing."

## Low-Riding Denim

Stars like **GWYNETH PALTROW** wear stretch versions of low-cut jeans slung under their bumps, often with a long fitted tunic." This is the sort of easy outfit that looks good without trying," says Hoppus. "Basic, basic pieces, but the shoes are making it."

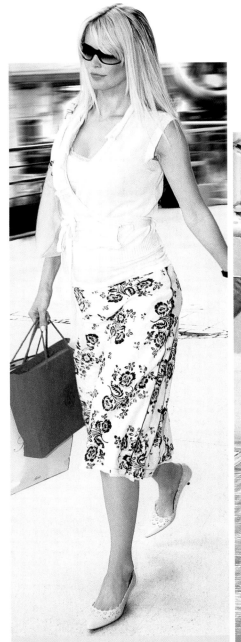

## Expandable Pieces

Wrap tops—like this knit version that **CLAUDIA SCHIFFER** layers over a cotton camisole and a print skirt—are ripe with potential. "A wrap is great," says Lange, "because it's adjustable through the whole nine months. You just tie it higher as your bump starts growing."

## Open-Jacket Policy

Stars started a trend by mixing in a lot of their prematernity clothes, even if the pieces couldn't be buttoned. "It's great to wear one of your favorite jackets, and just leave it open, like **SARAH JESSICA**'s doing here," says Hoppus. "It helps you feel like your old self."

## Instant Glam

The right accessories can glamorize a basic stretch dress. With her blossomy bag, Chanel ballet flats, and shades, **CATHERINE ZETA JONES** storms through an airport in a blaze of bump glory. "It's a very movie-star look," says Lange, "but easy to emulate."

"You do lose control, and it's quite a shock....You ask yourself, What am I going to do with this body?"

–UMA THURMAN
ON HER PREGNANCY

# red carpet mamas

A decade ago, the phrase "maternity glamour" simply didn't compute.
**Things, quite noticeably, have changed.**

**Madonna paved the way,** but the era of serious bump glam really began when a very pregnant **Sarah Jessica Parker** wore a swingy, white, empire-waist Narciso Rodriguez dress to a 2002 premiere—and managed to outshine, well, everyone. The impact on normal-person maternity style was immediate. Patrick McMullen, the well-known New York City party photographer, reported a sharp increase in chic pregnant Manhattanites "on the town." Most, he said, were "dressed to kill and camera-ready." In a city that normally feeds on weightier gossip, the hot rumor was that Manolo Blahnik had designed special, extra-comfy, kitten-heel shoes just for Sarah Jessica's swollen feet.

"The stars' willingness to step out onto the red carpet has made a huge difference," says Skye Hoppus, who's dressed moms-to-be **Courteney Cox** and **Reese Witherspoon**. "It's given other women the sense that, 'Hey, I can really look good.' " Of course, few expectant moms have the perfectly toned arms of SJP, or her relatively compact bump, but that doesn't mean they shouldn't try a slinky jersey gown or a strapless dress, says Liz Lange, who's worked with celebrities from **Uma Thurman** to **Julianne Moore**: "Many women think, 'Strapless? When I'm so big and fleshy? No way.' But when your belly's so huge, your arms actually look pretty good by comparison." Showing some skin can make you feel beautiful, she says. "I tell women not to forget that feeling sexy and sensual is what pregnancy is all about. I mean, isn't sex what got them there in the first place?"

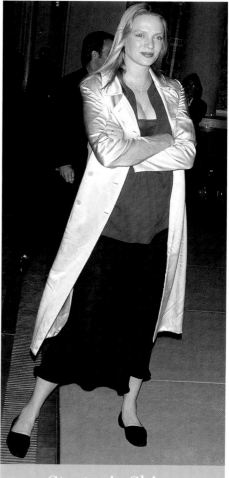

### Strategic Shine

**UMA THURMAN** starts with a low-key look (a loose tunic, a simple skirt, sensible loafers) then gives it star quality by throwing on a satin coat. "If you own a dressy trench," says Lange, "adapt it for your pregnancy."

### Regal Cuts

For big-event bump glamour, celebrities often go for a simple gown with an empire waist or a waistless trapeze style—like **DEBRA MESSING**'s chiffon Elie Saab gown. With its gold-embroidered bodice, it gives her the sort of power and dignity once missing from maternity style. "Very Greek goddess," says Lange.

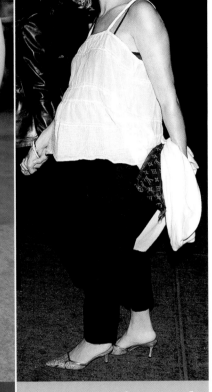

"In the '90s, pregnant celebrities hid out for nine months and just quietly had a baby. You certainly didn't see them at the Oscars. It's a different world now."

**—MATERNITY-WEAR DESIGNER LIZ LANGE**

## Feminine Color

Though most maternity "occasion" dresses are still safely black, **CYNTHIA NIXON** successfully risks girly pink. "When you're not feeling pretty because of your bulk," says Hoppus, "you want to add some feminine color, even if it's just a scarf around your neck."

## Daywear After Dark

**SARAH JESSICA PARKER** layers a sheer Marni apron top over a black bra for a radical-but-cool evening look. "She's broken all the rules," says Hoppus, "But it works." (While pregnant, SJP wore the same top combo on *Sex and the City*, paired with tight shorts and stilettos!)

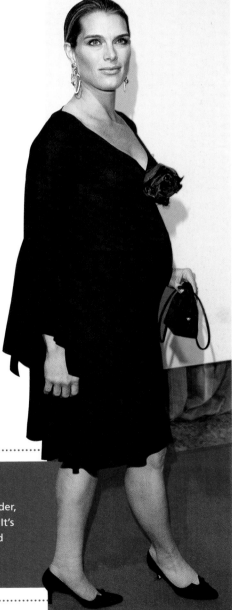

## Unapologetic Sexiness

If you think it's inappropriate for moms-to-be to smolder, please don't look at this photo of **BROOKE SHIELDS**. "It's a classic look, and so beautiful," says Hoppus. "If she'd worn her hair down, it wouldn't have worked so well. It's largely about the cleavage."

# four bumps, four styles

## REESE WITHERSPOON
### *chic traditional*

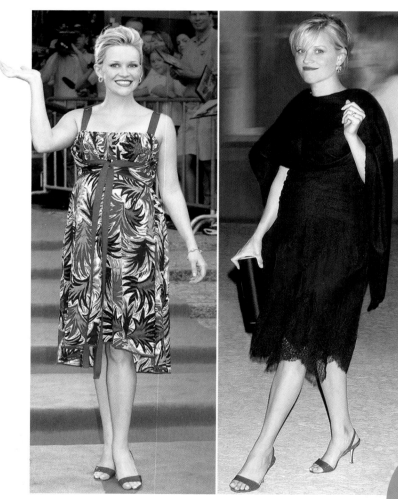

"Sometimes I felt like I was smuggling beach balls."
—REESE WITHERSPOON

✻ **BUMP STYLE:** A designer take on retro-'50s. A Southern lady, Reese wasn't about to waddle around the Santa Monica pier in a belly-baring tube top. Her key look was a flowy empire-waist dress in either classic black (above, right) or white (Prada, right) or a preppy print (custom-fit Missoni, above left).

✻ **STRATEGIES:** To deal with her new megabosom, Reese chose dresses with wide shoulder straps and skin-baring necklines. A disproportionate bust trapped in a high neck-line can make petite women like Reese look top-heavy—and ready to keel over.

✻ **TRADEMARKS:** Feminine ribbon details and her sexy red slingback mules—delicate enough to offset her bulk. As you can see, she rarely ventured out in public without them.

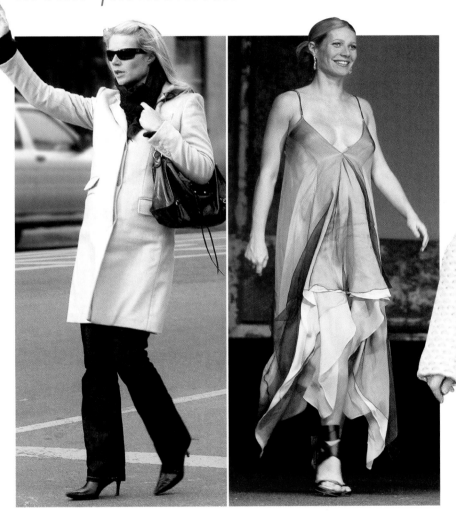

> "Gwyneth was just a beautiful, classy, hip mom-to-be. She encompassed everything that women want to be when they're pregnant."
> —CHILDISH DESIGNER SKYE HOPPUS

# GWYNETH PALTROW
*urban fashionista*

✳ **BUMP STYLE:** Being pregnant seemed to revitalize Gywneth's fashion sense (she also took a break from a joyless macrobiotic diet, gorging on grilled cheese sandwiches, which may have helped her mood). Clearly into her new body, she alternated classic basics (above, left) with more flamboyant pieces—from a cool turtleneck dress with an almost Elizabethan collar and cuff treatment (right) to a Stella McCartney chiffon gown (above, right).

✳ **STRATEGIES:** Gwyneth adapted a lot of non-maternity clothes (this clearly expandable sweater dress, for example) to avoid that predictable pregnancy look.

✳ **TRADEMARKS:** Her stretchy low-rise jeans. A proponent of the jeans-under-belly approach, Gwyneth often wore custom-made vintage-style jeans with three-button flares (right) from Los Angeles label Childish, which later added a version to their line.

# CATHERINE ZETA-JONES
*power glamour*

✳ **BUMP STYLE:** Catherine's formula throughout her pregnancies has been dead simple—all-black, all the time. Or, more accurately, all-black except when it's time to win an Oscar in chocolate-brown Versace (below right, at the 2003 Academy Awards). She keeps the statement strong and innovatively fabulous, varying textures (satin, velvet, feathers) if not color.

✳ **STRATEGIES:** Though black has become a bit passé in celebrity bumpland, it still dominates most maternity designers' "special event" lines for the obvious reason—you look approximately 10 percent smaller in it.

✳ **TRADEMARKS:** High-glam accessories—giant scarves (left), crystal-studded bags and ankle-strap sandals (below, left), and coveted gold figurines.

"Catherine is a throwback 'movie star,' so black really worked. Some cute peasant top just wouldn't make sense on her."

**—NOM'S JENNIFER NOONAN**

> "Katie's main concern was to have a happy baby. She didn't have that preoccupation with self—and that's what I most admire."
>
> **–KATE'S MOM, GOLDIE HAWN**

# KATE HUDSON
## *california bohemian*

✳ **BUMP STYLE:** Kate, who happily ballooned from 112 to 172 pounds during her pregnancy, adopted a cool, comfort-driven approach with zero concern about baring her belly. She loved simple stretch pieces (above, right), but pulled out all the stops for big events (in Chanel at the Venice Film Festival in 2003, right). Her boho look wasn't for everyone—an *Us Weekly* survey found that women far preferred Reese Witherspoon's more conservative style—but Skye Hoppus gives Kate major cred: "She's the perfect example of the modern, hip, young mom, truly celebrating her pregnancy. She really put it out there, and she didn't care."

✳ **STRATEGIES:** Kate had vowed to wear heels throughout her pregnancy, but often relied on her cozy, increasingly unhip Uggs (above, left).

✳ **TRADEMARKS:** Aforementioned belly, irrepressible enthusiasm

# "I WILL WORK HARD, I WILL KILL MYSELF, BUT NOBODY CAN SEPARATE ME FROM MY BABY. "

—UMA THURMAN
ON BRINGING HER INFANT SON TO HER MOVIE SET

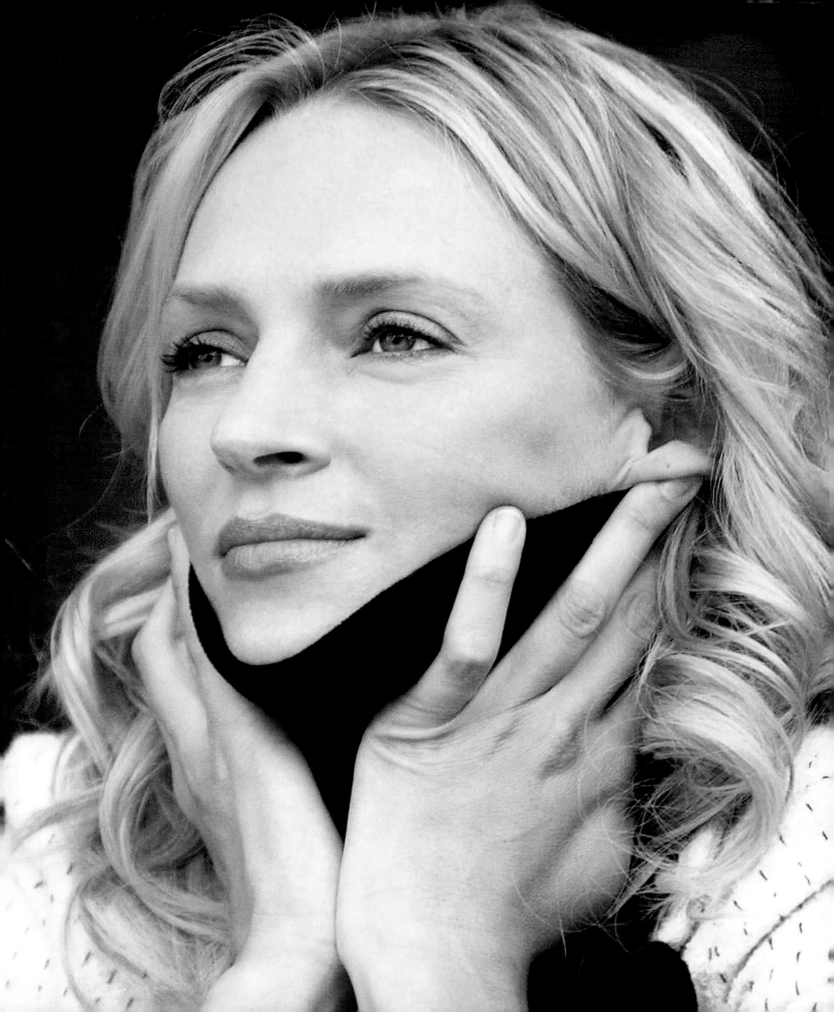

# chapter 12

# YOUR AGE STYLE

You'll never catch thirtysomething Jennifer Garner in a baby-doll dress that would flatter only a baby or a doll. Kirsten Dunst has wisely declared she's too young for diva gowns ("I want to look as much like myself as I can.") Both these stars know that—even in a world where teenagers wear tweeds and fortysomething Demi Moore is determinedly wrinkle-free—there's still some truth to the notion of "dressing your age." The key factor is trendiness. If you're under 30 or so, we'd be disappointed if you weren't testing trend limits. (Everyone has to wear feathers at least once.) But after that, it's probably time to become more discriminating and wistfully pack away those zebra-print short-shorts for your children to inherit. As the Lion King would say, it's the Circle of Life.

"Liv wants to find an outfit that makes a statement—and then have fun."

—MARY ALICE STEPHENSON, LIV TYLER'S STYLIST

# your teens

You're experimenting with **your style identity.** But is "preschooler" or "middle-aged broad" really the look you're after?

**Teenage celebrities, like puppies,** can get away with pretty much anything, especially when they're not in rehab. "Youth and money can be a powerful combination when it comes to fashion," says Jennifer Rade, who's styled **Avril Lavigne** and other MTV mini-moguls. "I love the way the **Olsen twins** take advantage of that. They'll take a really expensive Chanel blazer and throw it with sweatpants, and it just works." But being a millionaire teen can suck in its own way, says celebrity stylist Jill Swid: "When you're only 15, and you already own four Prada bags, what do you have to look forward to?"

Even Prada-less teens—inspired by stars like the Olsens and **Natalie Portman**, and increasingly turned-off by **Britney Spears**'s bare-midriff trashiness—are craving more sophistication, says Sara Rogers, teenage trend expert at the Mall of America in Bloomington, Minnesota: "You didn't use to see girls buying pencil skirts to wear to high school. This generation is so privileged—there's just an impatience to grow up." Tricky, that. Take sophistication too far with, say, a retro tweed skirt-suit and, suddenly, you're in old-person drag (unless you keep the suit playful by wearing it with a tee). On the flipside, too many girlish bows, and your look skews "Little Orphan Annie." But, at this age, so what? Even if you commit a fashion "don't," it's far better to experiment than to be a bore.

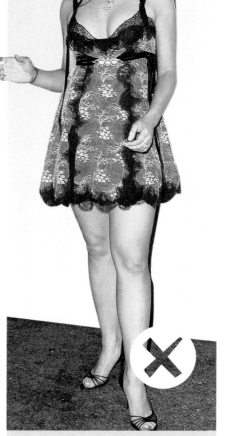

LINDSAY LOHAN

**Too Young: Doll Clothes**

Fashion victim alert! A baby-doll dress looks ridiculous on anyone over the age of six. This one is saying: "I am a wittle girl, even though I have enormous breasts."

## Miniskirts

A quintessential teen look: Cute, trendy, and sexy without drifting into tragic Britney territory. Graphic '80s accessories, like Lindsay's apple-green bag, edge it up.

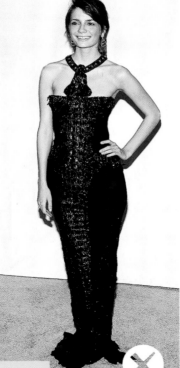

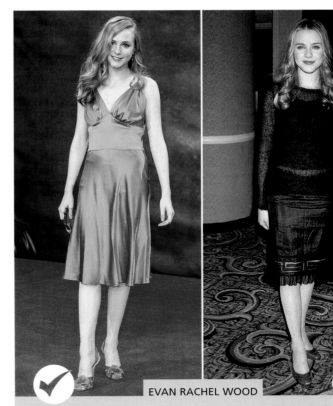

**MISCHA BARTON**

**TENDER DRESSES**
When you're still technically "carefree," a flowy wisp of a dress looks right.

**TOO OLD: STIFF GOWNS**
Why is Mischa dressing like an ex–Vegas showgirl on a Carnival Cruise?

**EVAN RACHEL WOOD**

**MTV COLOR**
Young skin can handle brights, and Evan's working it, down to the shoes.

**TOO OLD: LAWYER CHIC**
In sober pumps, she seems to be in negotiations to become an old fart.

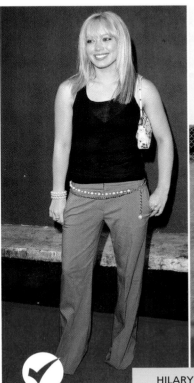

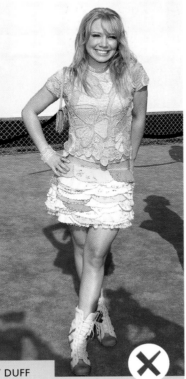

**HILARY DUFF**

**TRENDIFIED BASICS**
Hilary gives a clean look playful twists with a patterned bag and pearls.

**TOO YOUNG: TODDLER STYLE**
It is possible to be too cute. This outfit has since been confined to a crib.

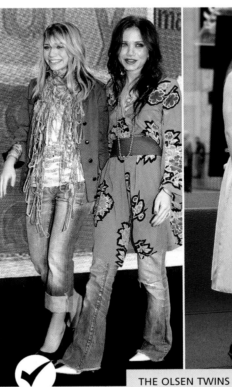

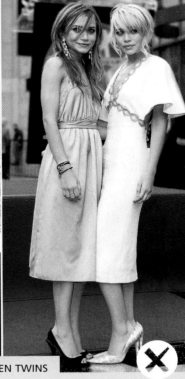

**THE OLSEN TWINS**

**JEANS 'N' TOPS**
Overly "ladylike" teens can seem alien. Denim brings them down to earth.

**TOO OLD: MOM'S SHOES**
Attempts to pull off high fashion flop when your shoes are clearly too big.

# the twenties

**It's freedom time.** The ideal vibe: Experimental, young, but sophisticated enough to get bumped up to first class.

**The 20s aren't entirely lighthearted**—not when you're weighed down with college debt, career angst, and unwanted overtures from guys who still think Dave Matthews is "sweet." But you're still really flexible on the style front, and, as long as you work with your body, few pieces are inappropriate, at least outside the office. Miniskirts. Supertight jeans. Vintage '40s blouses. You even have a fighting chance of looking cute in culottes.

To spout a fashion truism, it really is how you put it all together. Load on trends too giddily, and your clothes shriek "immaturity." Go too timeless and stiff—as **Scarlett Johansson** did recently in a black dress whose severity recalled the corpse of Eva Peron—and you can seem joylessly old. "I imagine when some of these girls are 35, they'll look back on those photographs and say, 'Oh my god, I was so young and beautiful. Why did I do that to myself?'," says celebrity stylist Jennifer Rade. "You really want to balance the two extremes."

Even **Eve**, a renowned risktaker, is working towards that goal in her later 20s, says her stylist Erin Hirsh. "Eve's taste is getting more and more refined. And she gets more attention when she goes for a subdued glamour look. That's when people really notice."

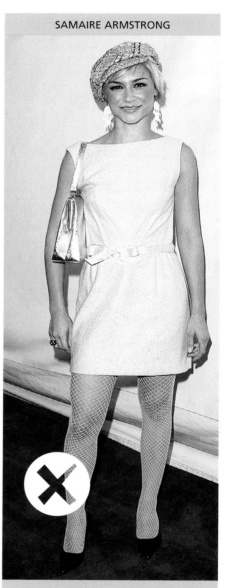

SAMAIRE ARMSTRONG

## Trend Sophisticate

Hip yet elegant is always a good mix: This dress combines a brash, retro-'80s color scheme with the delicacy of silk. Samaire softens its edges even further with a romantic locket.

## Too Young: Trend Victim

Once upon a time, all of these items, from the skull earrings to the newsboy cap, were hot. But even then, wearing them simultaneously—with clown makeup—was not.

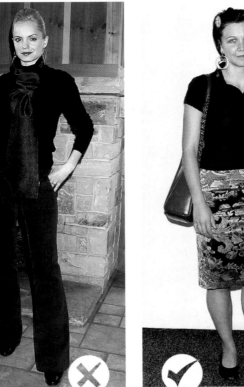

MENA SUVARI

**CAFFEINATED COLOR**
A fuchsia party dress gives Mena that "amped to stay up all night" look.

**TOO OLD: UPTIGHT BLACK**
"I am your German real-estate agent! My dog, Frieda, died! I hate you!"

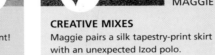

MAGGIE GYLLENHAAL

**CREATIVE MIXES**
Maggie pairs a silk tapestry-print skirt with an unexpected Izod polo.

**TOO OLD: MUMMIFIED FORMALITY**
For reasons known only to herself, she pays tribute to Nancy Reagan.

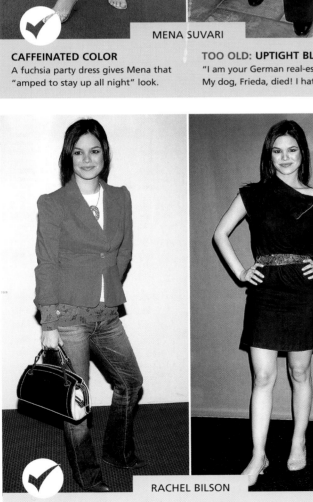

RACHEL BILSON

**CROPPED JACKETS**
Rachel looks put-together in a curve-hugging jacket layered over tees.

**TOO YOUNG: CUTESY SACKS**
A shapeless dress, and the least sultry shoes ever, make her seem childish.

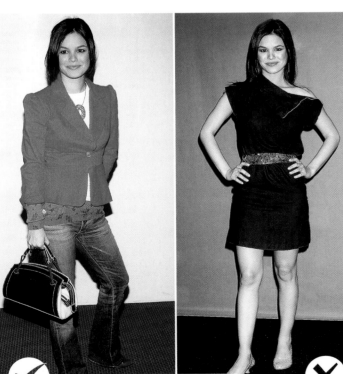

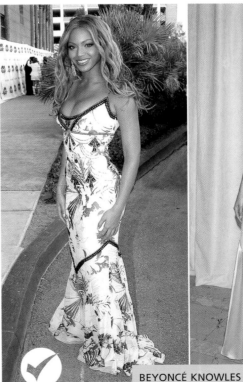

BEYONCÉ KNOWLES

**FLIRTY GOWNS**
If you have to wear a full-length gown, go for a soft, sexy, chiffon slip dress.

**TOO OLD: FRUMPY GOWNS**
Did Beyoncé borrow this geriatric dress from the Empress of Stuffiness?

# the thirties

**Your style is evolving**—except when (just like the stars) you suffer from temporary fashion insanity.

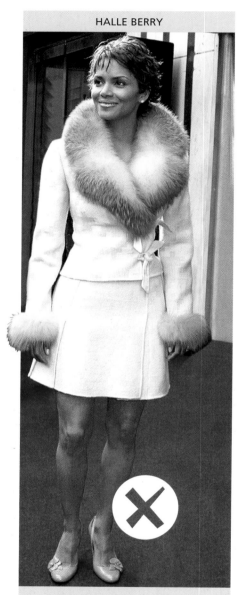

HALLE BERRY

### Too Old: Rodeo Drive Fur

On Halle, an enormous fur collar with matching cuffs says "movie star." On normal people, it can easily say, "ostentatious society lady with cheesy taste and a yappy Pekinese."

### Glam Suits

Halle, who's worn her share of grande-dame gowns, lets down her hair in a Dolce & Gabbana suit, the sort of powered-up classic that's ideal for your 30s.

**Entering your 30s can be a real relief.** Getting dressed is easier once you've begun to work out your formula and can rely on at least a few tried-and-true looks. You no longer roll your eyes at the phrase "investment buy." There's still room in your wardrobe for trends, but not at the expense of your dignity. (Ankle boots with skirts? Not a mistake you're willing to make again.).

Celebrities go through the same transition, says Jennifer Rade, who works with **Angelina Jolie**, a mother who recently turned 30: "Angie's definitely moving toward more classic pieces, a lot more skirts. I don't think she would have worked a floral Collette Dinnigan dress back when she was still with **Billy Bob Thornton** and wearing tons of leather." Rade says Angelina is even more selective about trends now: "If I showed her a baby-doll dress, she'd probably ask me if I'd had a concussion." Angelina is more likely to keep her look current with voguish separates, such as a metallic capelet that she recently wore over jeans and a tank (with her toddler Maddox in tow). And though she still wears a fair bit of color, she chooses subdued shades found in nature because they're more flattering, says Rade. "She doesn't wear neon pink, for example, but she might try a pretty olive."

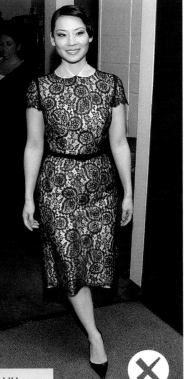

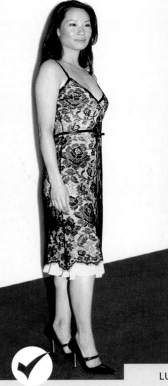

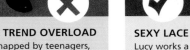

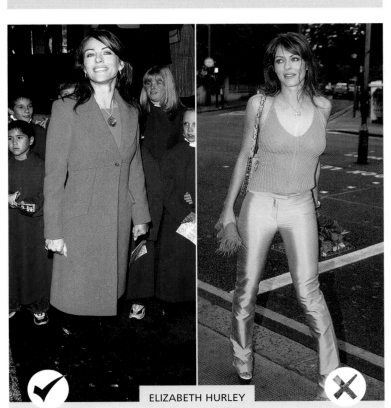

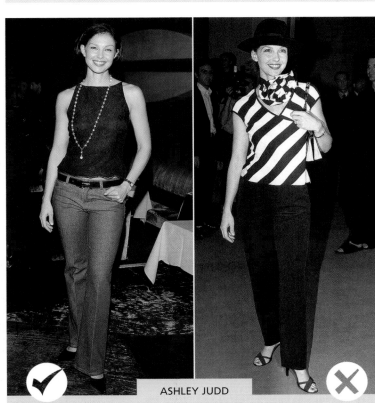

✔ REBECCA ROMIJN ✖

**TREND SELECTIVITY**
Rebecca zeros in on just one twist—bright shoes—to tweak a quiet look.

**TOO YOUNG: TREND OVERLOAD**
After being kidnapped by teenagers, Rebecca escapes in their cast-off clothes.

✔ LUCY LIU ✖

**SEXY LACE**
Lucy works a ladylike look that reveals enough skin to avoid the *old*-lady look.

**TOO OLD: PRUDISH LACE**
Lace plus a Peter Pan collar, plus tight shellacked hair? Way too governess.

✔ ELIZABETH HURLEY ✖

**POWER COLOR**
Mix up neutral separates with a jolty coat. You can always take it off.

**TOO YOUNG: NEONS**
Sexy—if your goal is to time-travel to 1980 and get carded at a roller disco.

✔ ASHLEY JUDD ✖

**STREAMLINED PIECES**
To move away from girlish, limit the frou-frou and go for cleaner lines.

**TOO OLD: RETIREE CHIC**
A matchy Ashley, fresh from winning "best dressed" at her local bingo hall.

# the forties

**What works:** Tailored pieces and subtle slinkiness. What doesn't: Anything your daughter wants you to give back *right now*.

**The 40s are really just an extension** of your 30s. The notion that you're supposed to shuffle off into a fashion netherworld of slacks and mushroom-appliqué sweaters is completely dead. At this age, it's really about further refining your 30s look, using all the knowledge about dressing your body that you've picked up over the years through trial and error. Work the formula—then, judiciously, shake it up. "One of the dangers is that you can get too styled," says **Uma Thurman**'s stylist Jill Swid, who also works with a number of high-powered female executives in New York City. "You don't walk out of the house anymore without being perfectly styled. People don't see your personality, your character. They just see your uniform."

When it's time to shake it up, however, don't rebel against consistency in that erratic **Sharon Stone** way, and suddenly wear a see-through corset to your kid's choir recital. (We all have a responsibility not to scar young psyches.) If a trend arrives that clicks for you, pick up a new piece but don't over-indulge. The simplest refresher strategy of all, says Mary Alice Stephenson, former fashion director at *Harper's Bazaar*, is accessories: "For older women, shoes and bags tend to be the quick fashion fix. It's just easier psychologically to splurge on a trendy purse than a trendy dress."

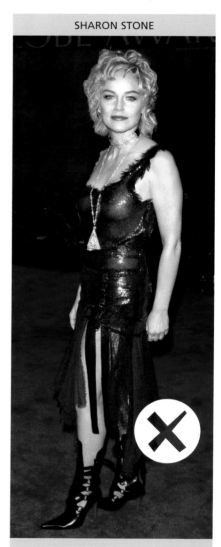

SHARON STONE

## Too Young: Bondage

This sadistically unflattering dress, or whatever you want to call it, wouldn't look good on anyone, except maybe a 21-year-old model at a fashion photo shoot involving panthers. And the panthers would have to wear very tight blindfolds so this garment wouldn't scare them.

## Ageless Denim

If you're more or less in shape, you can't go wrong in a well-cut pair of jeans, heels, and a great jacket—like Sharon's tweedy Chanel. (Wear a longer jacket if you're not that crazy about your hips.)

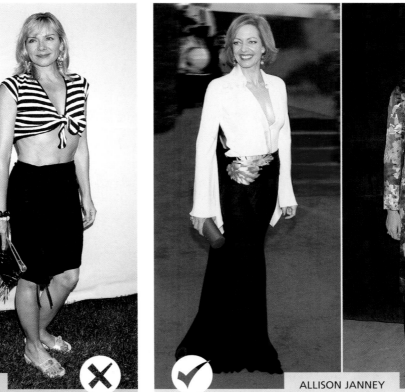

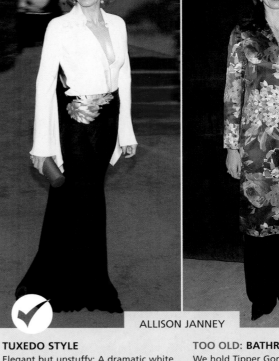

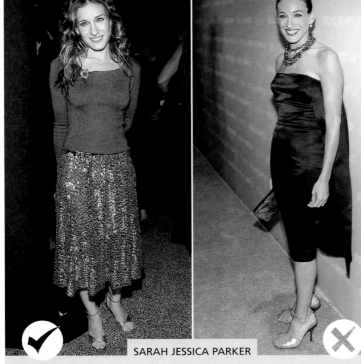

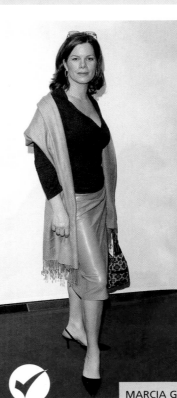

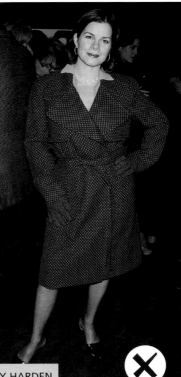

KIM CATTRALL

**CLEAVAGE**
If you've still got it, flaunt it tastefully in a vintage glam silk dress.

**TOO YOUNG: MIDRIFF**
Kim's audition for *Survivor: Gilligan's Island* goes poorly.

ALLISON JANNEY

**TUXEDO STYLE**
Elegant but unstuffy: A dramatic white shirt with a killer black skirt.

**TOO OLD: BATHROBE STYLE**
We hold Tipper Gore responsible for the unfortunate frock-coat look.

SARAH JESSICA PARKER

**JUST ENOUGH SHINE**
SJP subdues sparkle with a soft gray sweater, a smart move at any age.

**TOO OLD: SOCIETY-LADY CLICHÉS**
That cape's a bit "stately" for anyone younger than 110, don't you think?

MARCIA GAY HARDEN

**SHAPE-DEFINING SKIRTS**
A classic, tailored pencil skirt refines your look; leather keeps it sexy.

**TOO OLD: MATRONLY COATS**
Marcia looks prematurely unsvelte in a giant trench with bulkifying lapels.

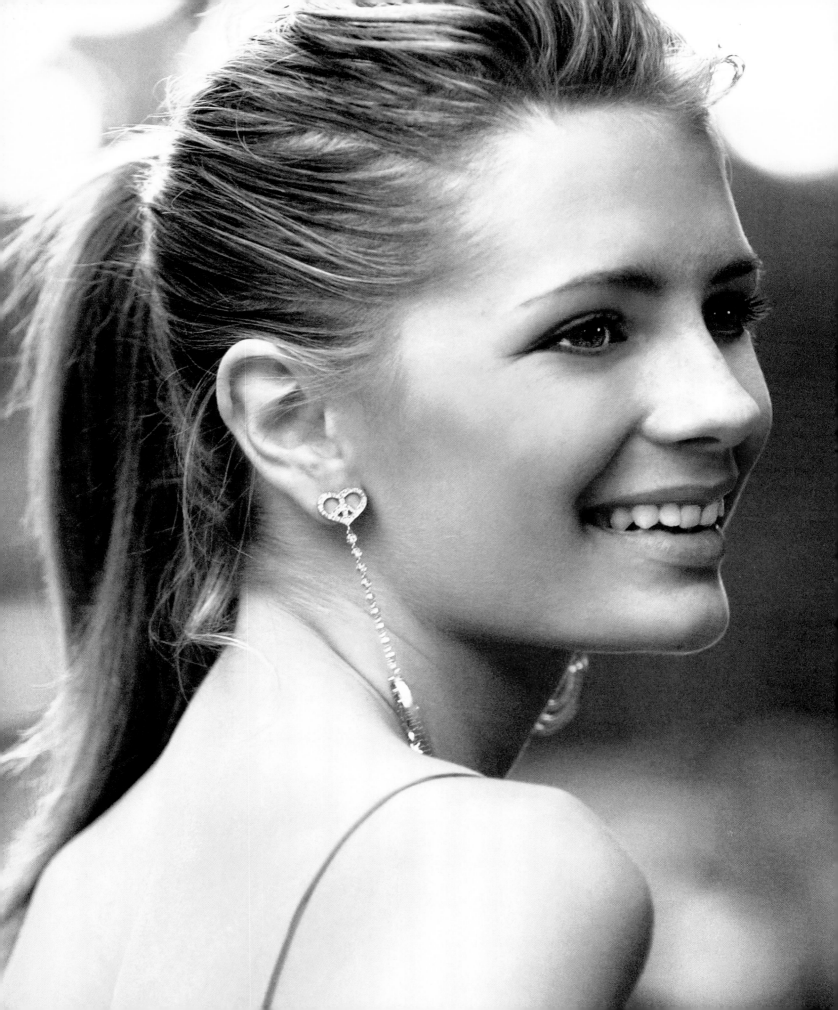

# "LORD KNOWS, MY STYLE IS GOING TO CHANGE AGAIN NEXT WEEK."

—MISCHA BARTON, 19, ON HER WORK-IN-PROGESS LOOK

# chapter 13

# SHOES & BAGS

"I definitely have a bit of a shoe fetish," Jennifer Aniston once admitted. "Men don't really notice women's shoes, but women wear them for each other." Men don't notice bags, either, or realize that shoes and bags have complex relationships that could fill the pages of a *Gone With the Wind*–size novel. A certain gold clutch, for example, might seem perfectly happy with matching slingbacks one weekend, only to be spotted dancing with some badass boots the next. Accessories can be mated so freely that such random combos often click. But to look as consistently turned out as your average Olsen twin, you need to think like a celebrity stylist, who might spend hours choosing the right mix to sex up a suit, or pacify a ruffled dress. Don't have hours? Here's the crash course.

"Our ability to accessorize is what separates us from the animals."

–OLYMPIA DUKAKIS IN *STEEL MAGNOLIAS*

# matching accessories

Harmonizing your shoes with your bag is a little old-school, but this ladylike strategy still has its uses if you're going for **instant dressiness or traditional chic.**

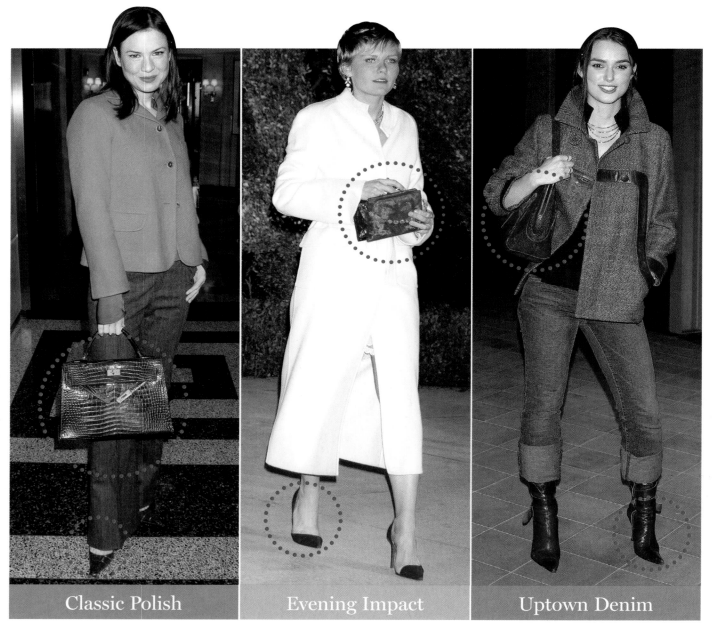

### Classic Polish

### Evening Impact

### Uptown Denim

Twinned accessories give tailored day looks a certain power. A crocodile Hermès Kelly bag plus refined croc heels, both in brown, complete **RENÉE ZELLWEGER** in a way Tom Cruise could not.

A color scheme simplified with matching accessories can help you make an even grander entrance. **KIRSTEN DUNST** allies a crimson brocade bag with her trademark cutaway Christian Louboutin pumps.

Jeans morph into sophisto-jeans with rich leather Chloe boots and a simpatico bag. **KEIRA KNIGHTLY** adds a leather-trimmed jacket to further distance herself from the world of poorly coordinated slobs.

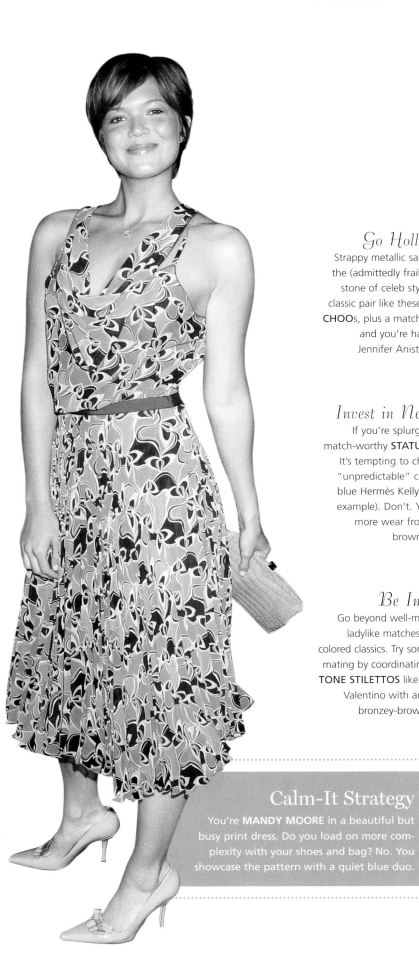

### Go Hollywood

Strappy metallic sandals are the (admittedly frail) corner-stone of celeb style. Get a classic pair like these **JIMMY CHOO**s, plus a matching bag, and you're halfway to Jennifer Aniston–ness.

### Invest in Neutrals

If you're splurging on a match-worthy **STATUS ITEM**. It's tempting to choose an "unpredictable" color (this blue Hermès Kelly Bag, for example). Don't. You'll get more wear from black, brown, or tan.

### Be Impolite

Go beyond well-mannered, ladylike matches of solid-colored classics. Try some sexier mating by coordinating **TWO-TONE STILETTOS** like these by Valentino with an olive or bronzey-brown clutch.

## Calm-It Strategy

You're **MANDY MOORE** in a beautiful but busy print dress. Do you load on more complexity with your shoes and bag? No. You showcase the pattern with a quiet blue duo.

# freestyle pairings

Off the red carpet, stylish stars often shun matchy-matchiness, and choose shoes and bags that **harmonize more loosely**—as long as they're in sync with the outfit's mood.

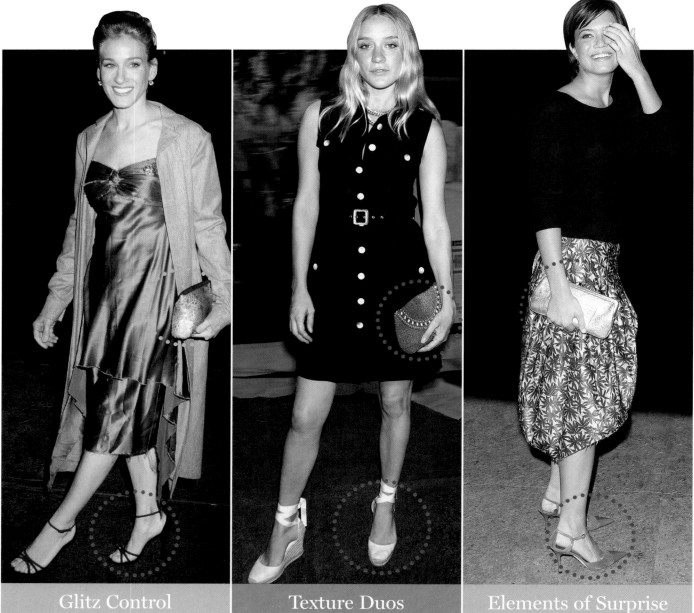

## Glitz Control

## Texture Duos

## Elements of Surprise

**SARAH JESSICA PARKER** uses unmatched accessories to restrain a Lanvin dress that doesn't need much more pizazz. A metallic snakeskin bag? Okay, but she cools it with matte black Balenciaga heels.

**CHLOE SEVIGNY** could have poshed up this shirtdress with matchiness, but goes a hipper route with espadrilles and a woven straw clutch that share nothing but texture and a laid-back vibe.

With this glammy skirt and a metallic Lambertson Truex bag, the obvious shoe choices would be black or silver. **MANDY MOORE** confounds our hidebound minds by picking a refreshing sage green.

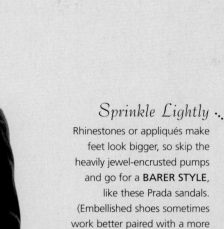

# CELEBRITY STYLIST TIP SHEET

## *Sprinkle Lightly*

Rhinestones or appliqués make feet look bigger, so skip the heavily jewel-encrusted pumps and go for a **BARER STYLE**, like these Prada sandals. (Embellished shoes sometimes work better paired with a more minimal bag—and vice versa.)

## *Use Pattern Wisely*

Boost a basic look with a **GRAPHIC BAG**, like this Coach hobo, but keep the shoes fairly basic too. Let us not to the marriage of a simple outfit and a patterned bag admit impediments.

## *Say No to Nurse*

White shoes tend to "pop" too much, overwhelming your other accessories, and ruining the line of your leg. Outside of the emergency ward, **IVORY OR PALE BEIGE** is usually more flattering.

## Internal Rhyme

It's not just about shoes and bags. In this more subtly coordinated look, **KIRSTEN DUNST**'s brown Chloe Silverado bag connects with the color of her belt. The boots are on their own.

# color play

**Think of accessories like makeup**—dabs of color that can bring out an outfit's beauty, or transform a snoresome look as quickly as lipstick wakes up a sleepy face.

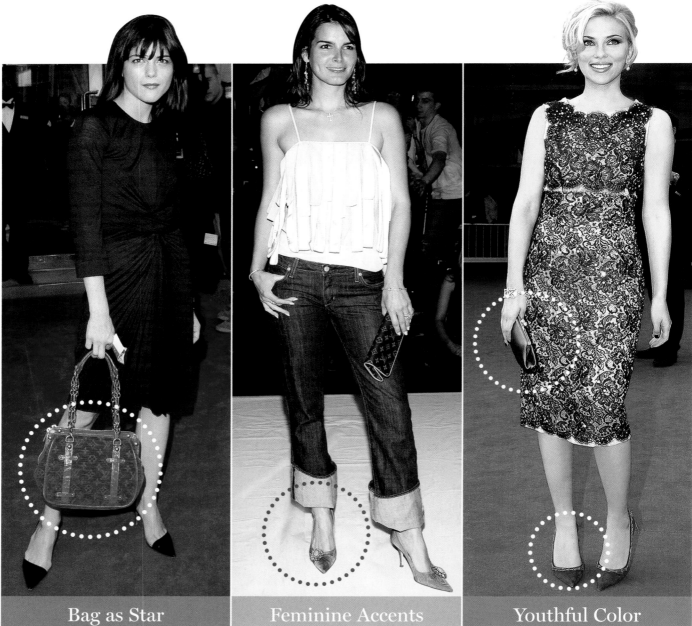

## Bag as Star

## Feminine Accents

## Youthful Color

Classically chic: carrying a bravura purse as a single hit of color. **SELMA BLAIR** indulges her red Louis Vuitton bag's ego by showcasing it against the neutral backdrop of a vintagey little black dress.

Brown isn't girlish. Black is rather stern. To romanticize jeans, consider the gentler colors. **ANGIE HARMON** de-tomboys her denim with daintily brooched dusty rose Jimmy Choo pumps.

If you wear any "mature" ladylike look with drab accessories, you can appear prematurely elderly. **SCARLETT JOHANSSON** uses blue and ruby pieces to prevent a gray lace dress from mildewing.

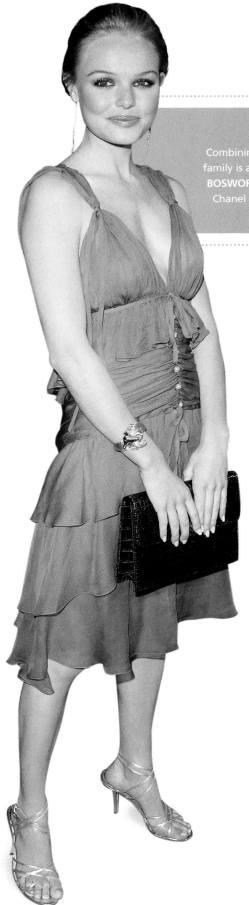

### Related Hues

Combining shades from the same color family is a subtly elegant strategy. **KATE BOSWORTH** inter-marries her lavender Chanel dress with pale mauve sandals and a profoundly purple bag.

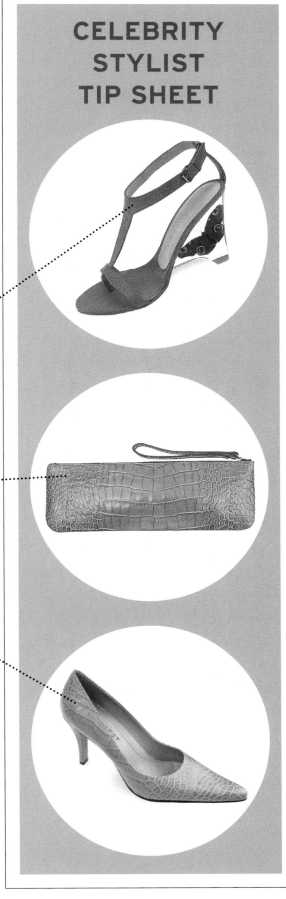

## Avoid "Stump Leg"

T-strap shoes can be risky (and not just for butterflies). A thick, brightly colored ankle strap like this "chops" off legs, and makes them look shorter. Look for **PALER, THINNER STRAPS**.

## Clutch Less

Do you really want to hold a clutch all night just to showcase your genius color sense? Choose one with a **WRIST STRAP**, like this Club Monaco number. Then you can actually carry a drink. Or two.

## Orange You Glad?

The easiest way to revive a sluggish wardrobe? Enthusiastically bright shoes. Even the most generic khakis will **KICK UP THEIR HEELS** if you give them heels like this.

# mood shifters

If you're tired of routinely pretty outfits or predictable glamour, use unexpected accessories to flip your look and give it a **whole new vibe**.

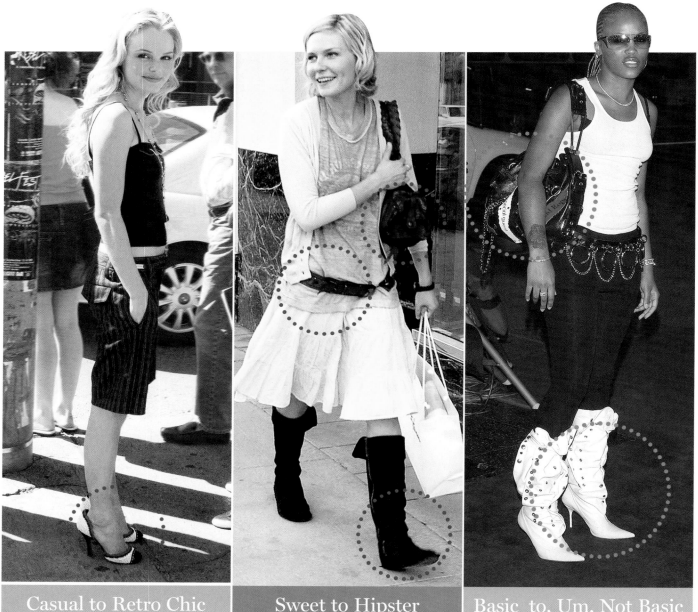

### Casual to Retro Chic

### Sweet to Hipster

### Basic to, Um, Not Basic

Striped shorts. A summery top. **KATE BOSWORTH** could have relaxed this cute look even further with blah slides, but twists it all the way to glamour with textured, '40s-ish D'Orsay pumps by Prada.

A useful trick: Contrasting feminine clothes with harder-edged accessories. **KIRSTEN DUNST** gives a pastel skirt a brutal crash course in urban reality (with the same accessories she's wearing on page 195.).

Remove all the accessories from this outfit and you're left with...a tank top and black leggings. **EVE** demonstrates the transformative power of accessories in her own inimitable ultra-glam way.

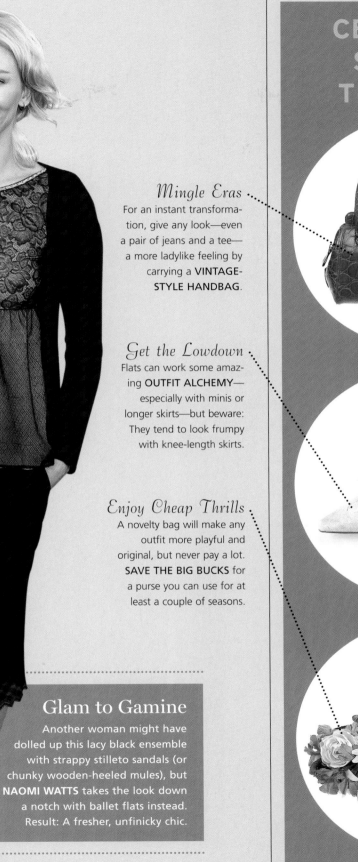

### Mingle Eras

For an instant transformation, give any look—even a pair of jeans and a tee—a more ladylike feeling by carrying a **VINTAGE-STYLE HANDBAG**.

### Get the Lowdown

Flats can work some amazing **OUTFIT ALCHEMY**—especially with minis or longer skirts—but beware: They tend to look frumpy with knee-length skirts.

### Enjoy Cheap Thrills

A novelty bag will make any outfit more playful and original, but never pay a lot. **SAVE THE BIG BUCKS** for a purse you can use for at least a couple of seasons.

### Glam to Gamine

Another woman might have dolled up this lacy black ensemble with strappy stiletto sandals (or chunky wooden-heeled mules), but **NAOMI WATTS** takes the look down a notch with ballet flats instead. Result: A fresher, unfinicky chic.

# make me over!

The wrong accessories can spoil an actually decent dress—or cheesify jeans. There's never just one right answer, but here's how we'd tweak some typical problem looks.

## PARIS HILTON

### PROBLEM:
### TACKY MATCHINESS

An arguably pretty, ribbon-tied dress gets cartoonish when forced to co-exist with overly coordinated accessories that rob it of its uniqueness. Matching shoes, maybe. Matching *ribbon* shoes? Overkill.

### SOLUTION:
### MINIMALIST GLAMOUR

Let that poor dress alone by surrounding it with simple gold accessories that don't compete for attention.

### *Quieter Bangle*
Keep some of the dress's colors in the bracelet...just not all of them.
CITRINE BY THE STONES

### *Fuzz-Free Bag*
Paris's fluffy purse is too cutesy. Sub in a crisp clutch with natural fur details.
KATE SPADE

### *Simpler Heels*
In ballerina shoes, Paris is performing a *faux pas de deux*. Better: restrained sandals. HOLLYWOULD

# JESSICA SIMPSON

## PROBLEM:
### FAILED FUNKINESS

This jeans outfit wants to be laid-back and even "edgy," but ends up looking sweet, meek, and kitschy due to a severe lack of earthiness. Too much white!

## SOLUTION:
### HELLO, BROWN

Import accessories with more warmth, texture, and toughness. (P.S. De-poof the hair—Jessica always looks cooler when she pulls it back into a ponytail.)

## Gutsier Scarf
Jessica's thin white scarf is too tuxedo—this untamed muffler has more soul. JOCELYN

## A Real Belt
We'd rather see Jessica in leather that looks like leather—minus all those chains.
JEAN PAUL GAULTIER

## Earthier Boots
A little less snow-bunny, a lot more funky. MUKLUK

## HILARY DUFF

### PROBLEM:
### PREDICTABILITY
When you're 17, it's a bit boring to accessorize a white suit with more white (down to your toenails)—especially if the pieces are as clunky as these.

### SOLUTION:
### CHIC COLOR
Go more Cameron Diaz—and play off the suit's simplicity with surprising accessories that mix graphic power with feminine delicacy.

### Non-Flintstones Jewelery
Lose the chunky Wilma necklace and add graceful earrings that work the new color scheme. WENDY MINK

### Joltier Bag
We'd replace that pale, lumpy pouch with this '80s clutch, jazzy but luxe. BOTTEGA VENETTA

### Unmellow Yellow Heels
Her shoes' bows are getting lost under those pants. These citrus sandals would peek out more boldly. BOTTEGA VENETTA

# CATHERINE ZETA-JONES

## PROBLEM:
### MIXED MESSAGES

It looks odd to wear a fancy black evening dress but haul around a hefty day bag. Catherine's other accessories also seem out-of-sync with the dress's mood.

## SOLUTION:
### A UNIFIED THEME

How about a more put-together, red-and-black strategy? A compact satin bag, more elegant shoes, and a necklace that takes advantage of that (non-daytime) cleavage.

### Sexier Stones

Turquoise is beautiful, but this onyx pendant has a higher glam quotient. DAVID AUBREY

### A Proper Evening Bag

Catherine's purse is just too big. This snazzy little guy has what it takes.
SALVATORE FERRAGAMO

### Dressier Shoes

A closed-toe shoe in black satin...yes, that's better.
RICKARD SHAH

# chapter 14

# STYLE PITFALLS

Look at poor **Christina Aguilera** over there. Not only is she wearing the world's droopiest cowl-neck dress, her feet have apparently become ensnared in badger traps. That's got to hurt. Christina isn't alone when it comes to celebrities who've fallen prey to bad fashion: They've been smothered in fur, cheesified by animal prints. Bulkifying metallic pieces have made the skinniest stars seem chunky. Even denim can turn treacherous when stylists try too hard to dress it up. Long story short: Too much *anything* messes up your look, especially if you wear it from head to toe. This doesn't mean you have to walk around sadly restrained—unshiny, unfluffy, unsexy, unzebra'd, unable to express yourself. The worst fashion of all is uptight fashion. Just remember: A little splendor goes a long way.

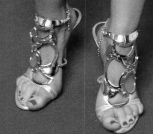

"I don't believe in the words *fashion faux pas*."

—CHRISTINA AGUILERA

# metallics

"Mousey" and "celebrity" don't really go together, which might explain why some stars overindulge in **high-gloss style**.

**"Celebrities are like magpies,"** *New York Observer* fashion expert Simon Doonan once said. "They're attracted to anything that *glints*." Magpies, of course, don't fly about in beak-to-claw metallic ensembles, while stars often swathe themselves in shine. Not a look to emulate, says **Angelina Jolie**'s style guru, Jennifer Rade: "If you wear anything head-to-toe—metallic, fur, denim, leather—you cross the line from fashion into something that's costumey and rather hard to take seriously."

Subdue shiny pieces by mixing in other separates in matte fabrics (wool, chiffon, jersey, even corduroy) or by showing enough skin to reassure people that you're not the heartless Tin Man from *The Wizard of Oz*. Metallic dresses, says Rade, are sexiest when they're sleeveless and simple: light-reflecting clothes tend to bloat you visually, so go for streamlined cuts (no excessive ruffles or draping). Choose thin, fluid fabrics that won't bulk you up the way silver leather does, for example. Finally, ixnay on the cheap gold lamé. It's just *too* shiny, says Rade. "Lamé should be reserved for music videos or drag queens."

## Fluidity

Metallic fabric looks prettiest when it's thin and flowy enough to skim your body without clinging. **MANDY MOORE** avoids overkill in a Calvin Klein halter that's half-molten and half-chiffon.

## Pitfall: Iceberg Chic

Stiff shiny fabrics can be cruel. Look what double-faced satin did to **SARAH JESSICA PARKER**, in a rigid, conical coat seemingly inspired by Mrs. Butterworth's unique bottom-heavy style.

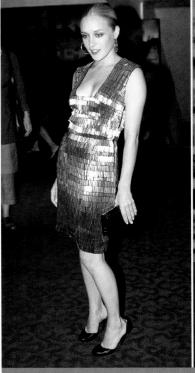

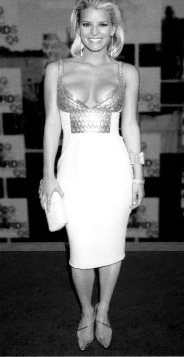

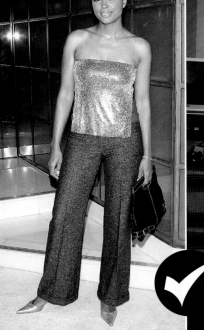

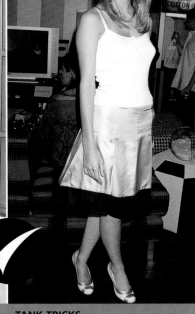

**CLEAN SHAPES**
Reflective fabric makes any look seem more complex, so go for a simple silhouette, like CHLOE SEVIGNY's sheath.

**SELECTIVE SHINE**
A restrained JESSICA SIMPSON limits herself to metallic details (often more elegant than full-length gloss).

**SOFT CONTRASTS**
When juxtaposed with tailored wool pants, AISHA TYLER's sequined top radiates more specialness.

**TANK TRICKS**
Like jeans, a tank top guarantees against overkill. MISCHA BARTON makes a seriously shiny skirt look summery.

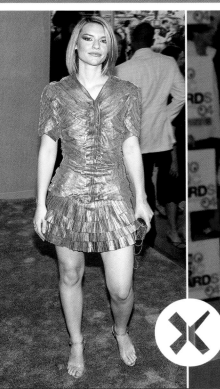

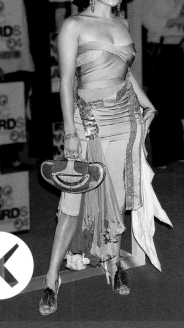

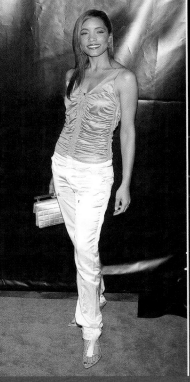

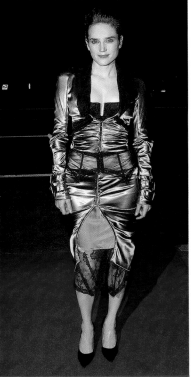

**PITFALL: CHUBBIFICATION**
Metallics already bulk you up—why add shoulder-pads and ruffles? Even superfit CLAIRE DANES looks lumpy here.

**PITFALL: GLAMOUR OVERDOSE**
J. Lo started with a few sequins, but soon she was shining nightly. Then she tried feathered shoes...and cowboy hats...

**PITFALL: HEAD-TO-TOE GLARE**
An hour after the event, MICHAEL MICHELLE used this tin-foil-esque outfit to bake more than 90 potatoes.

**PITFALL: CLINGY FIT**
In a tight metallic corset dress, a creased and crushed JENNIFER CONNELLY (literally) looks like a train wreck.

# wearing fur

**Real or faux, it says "luxury."** But when stars envelop themselves too exuberantly, it also says, "shapeless fluffy freak."

**Sensual, ladylike, mood-transforming,** fur is practically a synonym for glamour. And, while the practice of snatching coats from animals remains controversial for good reason, both high fashion and celebrities (even in balmy Los Angeles) have recently succumbed to its allure. Result: Half of Hollywood spent the winter looking fatter (at least in the shoulder area) thanks to a vogue for chubby fur stoles.

That's entirely avoidable, says Mary Alice Stephenson, celebrity stylist and the former fashion director of *Harper's Bazaar*: "The key is not to go overboard. There are a lot of fur options and technological advances that have eliminated the fluff factor." Among the best bets, she says, are sheared mink shrugs or bolero jackets: "I just find them more flattering than a full-on sable or fox coat." Not to mention more affordable. If you're on a tighter budget, she also suggests buying a vintage or flea-market fur (or recycling your mom's castoff) and having it sheared and retailored. "I also know some very chic New Yorkers," she says, "who've bought flea-market furs with yummy satin linings and just worn them inside out."

## Pitfall: Fur Overload

Overdo the warm 'n' fuzzy look and you can suddenly gain 100 pounds and spook small children. **ASHANTI**, apparently concerned her credit cards might get chilly, even adds a fur bag.

## Streamlined Luxury

A sleek sheared mink jacket wraps you in coziness with zero risk of blobbification. **KATE MOSS,** the essence of modern glamour, wears hers ultra-simply with a no-b.s. bright dress.

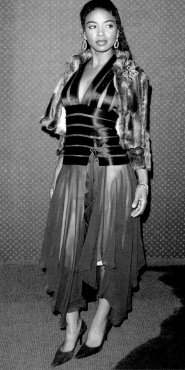 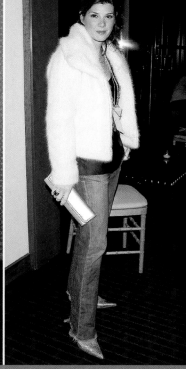 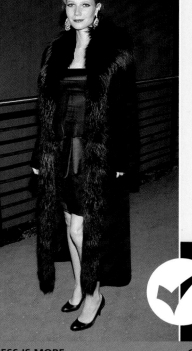 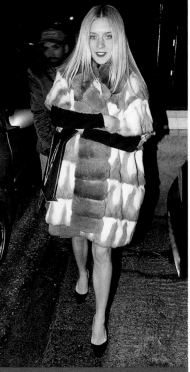

**VINTAGE GLAMOUR**
ANANDA LEWIS cozies up to retro in a cropped fur jacket, a less predictable look than a stole (below).

**DRESSED-DOWN OPULENCE**
Fur looks younger and less stodgy mixed with denim. MARISA TOMEI keeps things posh with metallic accessories.

**LESS IS MORE**
A fur collar and trim gives GWYNETH PALTROW's look grandeur without the bloat of a full fluffy coat.

**CLASSIC MINK**
Old-school simplicity makes it cooler than some self-consciously "designed" fur. ASHLEY OLSEN wears hers sheared.

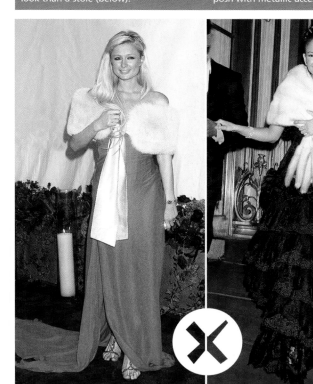 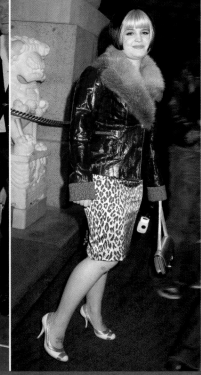 

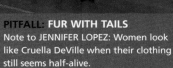

**PITFALL: DYED PELTS**
Even if it's fake, pink fur is decidedly cheesy. Not that PARIS HILTON would have it any other way...

**PITFALL: FUR WITH TAILS**
Note to JENNIFER LOPEZ: Women look like Cruella DeVille when their clothing still seems half-alive.

**PITFALL: FASHION-VICTIM FUR**
Leather, fur, leopard-print...KELLY OSBOURNE attempts to summarize the world of wildlife in one outfit.

**PITFALL: PATTERN**
CHLOE SEVIGNY wearing a furry backgammon board. If you turn it inside out, you can play Chinese Checkers.

# denim

Jeans are **endlessly versatile**. They give, give, give, and never take—so why do people do such unspeakable things to them?

You'd think something as basic as denim wouldn't have pitfalls. Does oxygen have pitfalls? Yet denim has been the undoing of some otherwise goof-free stars. The notion that jeans can be mixed with *anything* ("Hey, don't worry...you're dressing it down!") has led celebrities to pair them with some hideously over-elaborate "cute tops" (see "The Cute Top Hall of Shame," page 120), scary jackets, and ridiculous belts. And when a celebrity— or anyone, for that matter—falls for the more questionable types of "distressing," the jeans themselves become the problem.

"I don't like denim when the processing has been done too obviously and has zero organic quality," says stylist Jennifer Rade. "For instance, when a pair of jeans is bizarrely 'faded' on the butt or down the back of the thighs." Equally unsettling: any faded area that's been tinted that curious yellow shade which suggests you've just peed yourself. Darker (or even raw) denim with no special effects is generally the most sophisticated option.

Another Rade peeve: fake "holes" patched from inside the jeans with kitschy snowflake-patterned cotton. "To me, the whole point of denim is that it's casual and lived-in and real," she says. "If you're not going to keep the jeans part of your outfit natural, what's the point?"

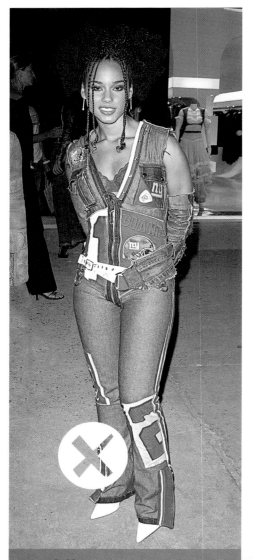

## Pitfall: "Customization"

Not many stars have the courage to turn to their stylists and say, "Make me look like a NASCAR racing car—except with more buckles and zippers." **ALICIA KEYS** gets victimized by the recent trend for one-of-a-kind, collaged-denim pieces.

## Dressed-up Denim

Classic jeans are a beloved outfit component because you can load on the glam and their intrinsic casualness (usually) protects you from "trying too hard." **EVE** gets it right.

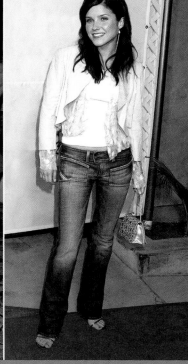

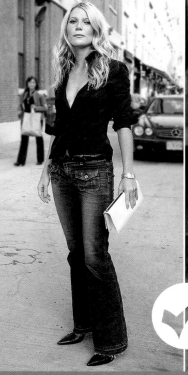

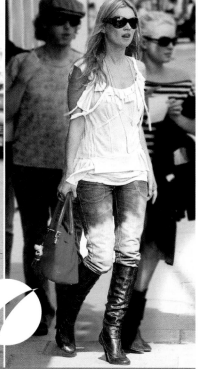

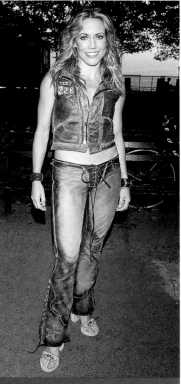

**EASYGOING CHIC**
As UMA THURMAN knows, a jean jacket makes any look—even a black pencil skirt—seem approachable and cool.

**LOW-KEY LAYERING**
Updated '70s-style Diesel jeans are a solid anchor for SOPHIA BUSH's subtle white-on-white-on-white layering.

**CLASSIC HOTNESS**
Adapt, if you dare, GWYNETH PALTROW's sexy formula: retro jeans, boots and a recklessly unbuttoned shirt.

**DIVA BOOTS**
Denim is the perfect foil for fashionista accessories. KATE MOSS works skinny boots and a cherry-red Birkin bag.

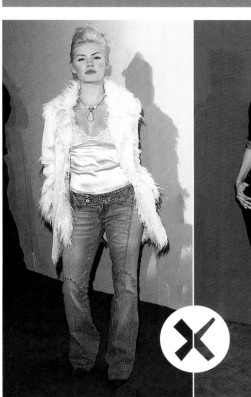

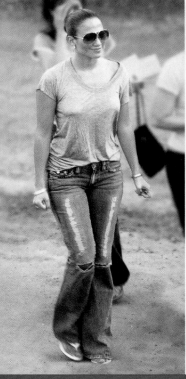

**PITFALL: GLITZ OVERLOAD**
ELISHA CUTHBERT was teetering safely on the edge of excess, then she went and Bedazzled her jeans.

**PITFALL: HEAD-TO-TOE BLUE**
Wearing denim top and bottom—or as a jumpsuit à la TYRA BANKS—always looks costumey. Even her mules are denim!

**PITFALL: IMPLAUSIBLE DISTRESSING**
JENNIFER LOPEZ demonstrates the dangers of trying to put your thighs through a paper shredder.

**PITFALL: OVER-PROCESSED DENIM**
Shortly after this photo was taken, SHERYL CROW's jeans were hospitalized "for exhaustion."

# showing skin

Remember Britney Spears's circa-1999 midriff? **That was then**, **this is now**. And the rules (and the erogenous zones) have changed.

**"Am I too daring?"** a certain megastar once wrote. "I ask this question with absolute sincerity because, in the last few months, several influential women have told me that I am. I have been accused of having terrible taste in clothes, of showing off too much, and of making vulgar use of my figure on a lot of social occasions."

**Britney Spears? Paris Hilton?** No, actually: Marilyn Monroe in an article she penned for *Modern Screen* magazine in 1952, which just underlines the fact that, in America, controversial "vulgarity" is as timeless as pearls.

While Paris is doing her best to carry on the tradition of daring (with occasional, unfocused help from **Tara Reid**), much of the country has adopted a more modest mood. Bare midriffs are passé. See-through tops, a coy novelty a few years ago, are seen less often. Teenagers are buying prom dresses so prim they practically have turtlenecks. For some, this latest wave of conservativism might seem restrictive, but, as stylist Jennifer Rade points out, it's also a chance to rediscover more subtly sexy parts of the body: "I personally love bare shoulders. And I have to say, when everyone's always wearing jeans, calves don't get enough love."

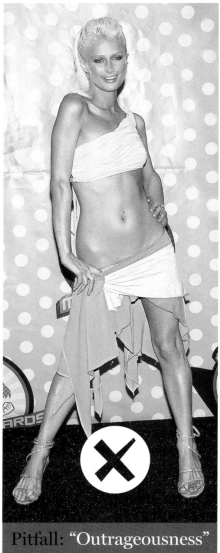

Pitfall: "Outrageousness"

If you're notably immodest, wrap a few turquoise scraps around yourself like **PARIS HILTON**, then try really hard to push them off your body.

## Leggy Fun

If you've got notable limbs, a mini (or minidress) works, especially if you avoid overexposure like **CAMERON DIAZ**, and stay a little more covered up top.

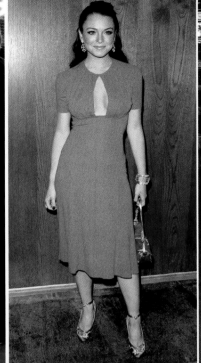 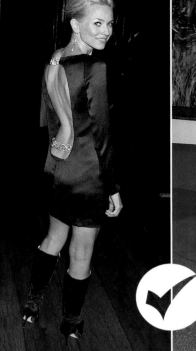 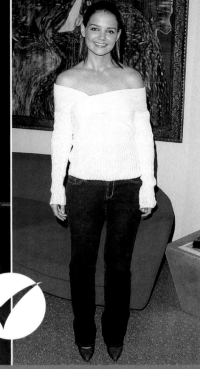

**STEALTH REVELATIONS**
A slit skirt is classically sexy, whether it's slit a few inches or—like CHARLIZE THERON's—a few miles.

**LADYLIKE CLEAVAGE**
LINDSAY LOHAN centers our attention with a keyhole neckline that's both racy and sophisticated.

**ALTERNA-SENSUALITY**
Who needs décolletage when you've got a back this beautiful? NAOMI WATTS showcases some little-seen curves.

**SHOULDERS, ANYONE?**
Off-the-shoulder style isn't restricted to gowns. KATIE HOLMES gives a white sweater the slip.

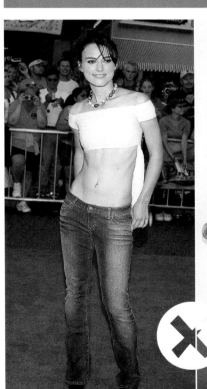 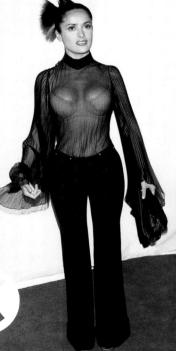 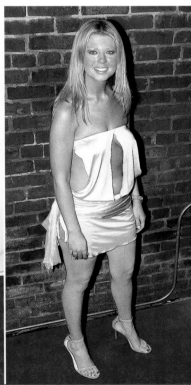 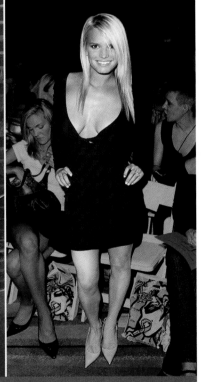

**PITFALL: ABS EXHIBITIONISM**
Do you get the feeling KEIRA KNIGHTLEY wants us to know she performs 14,000 sit-ups per day?

**PITFALL: SHEER INSANITY**
You know, that SALMA HAYEK sure has a nice body. Of course, that's just a guess.

**PITFALL: PATHOS**
In pale blue silk, TARA REID loosely interprets the refined, ladylike style of Jacqueline Kennedy Onassis.

**PITFALL: TROUBLING CLEAVAGE**
JESSICA SIMPSON can barely contain herself in a dress that does nothing to counteract gravity.

# animal prints

### The best ways to wear this somewhat uncontrollable look? **As classically as possible**—or dressed down with jeans.

**There's a dangerous amount of glamour** in one square inch of leopard-print. That hasn't stopped reckless stars from wearing it by the yard and looking just a bit insane. Animal prints, with few exceptions, tend to work best when they're used as sparingly as tattoo ink. The safest bet: a pair of shoes or a bag. If you want a larger dose of wildness, says celebrity stylist Mary Alice Stephenson, who works with **Liv Tyler**, a little leopard-print tank or camisole, for instance, can be a great layering piece. "I also like a leopard-print trench," she says. "Think '50s and lady-like. It doesn't work for me if the coat's too boxy, or complicated, or ultra-long. The animal print is really enough."

The best thing about these patterns: They claw their way back into fashion roughly every two years, so even if you contract a disorienting case of jungle malaria and overspend on spots, you'll eventually get your money's worth. "Store it in your closet," says Stephenson, "because sure enough, it will come back again."

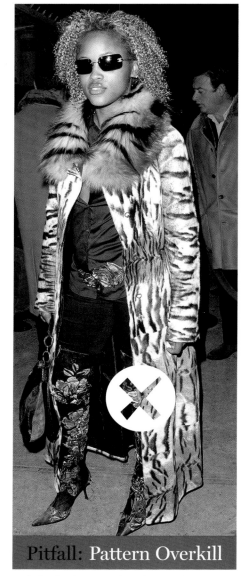

## Old-school Glamour

If you're going to invest in a leopard-print coat, a simple cut like **JENNIFER LOPEZ**'s classic balmacaan (with discreet, small-scale spots) is the way to go.

### Pitfall: Pattern Overkill

Animal prints are already complex enough without crazy fur collars and floral boots. **EVE** can (almost) pull this off, but it's not exactly what you'd call a soccer-mom look.

**CASUAL SWAGGER**
In strategically unglamorous jeans, GWEN STEFANI achieves a more relaxed mix than EVE (see opposite page).

**UNDERSTATEMENT**
AMBER VALETTA wears the leopard look gently in a sheer top that's not too in-your-face.

**SPOTTY DETAILS**
Often, animal prints work best as a single accessory hit like MENA SUVARI's pointy paw shoes.

**ENOUGH WITH THE LEOPARD!**
CLAUDIA SCHIFFER, showcasing a zebra skirt against a black turtleneck and boots, gets extra marks for originality.

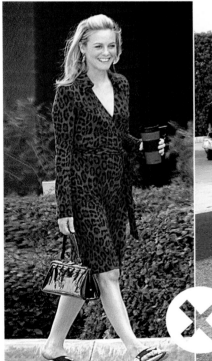

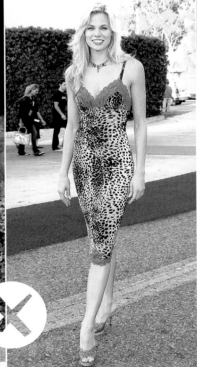

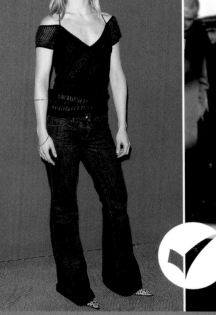

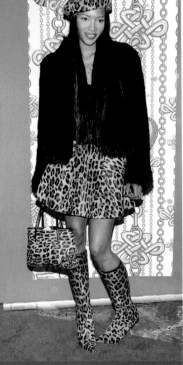

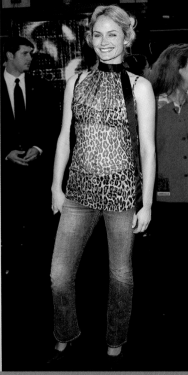

**PITFALL: UNNATURAL COLOR**
ALICIA SILVERSTONE in dyed leopard, a kitschy look that's only super-super-cute on Aerosmith.

**PITFALL: BOUDOIR BLENDS**
BROOKE BURNS's leopard and pink-lace slip dress has a corny "sexiness" that's better left to silly lingerie.

**PITFALL: BEASTLY SHINE**
With a few exceptions, such as wet walruses, animals aren't shiny. VIVICA FOX overdoes it in a metallic gown.

**PITFALL: MEASLES**
NAOMI CAMPBELL looks unwell. We recommend plenty of fluids and fewer matching berets.

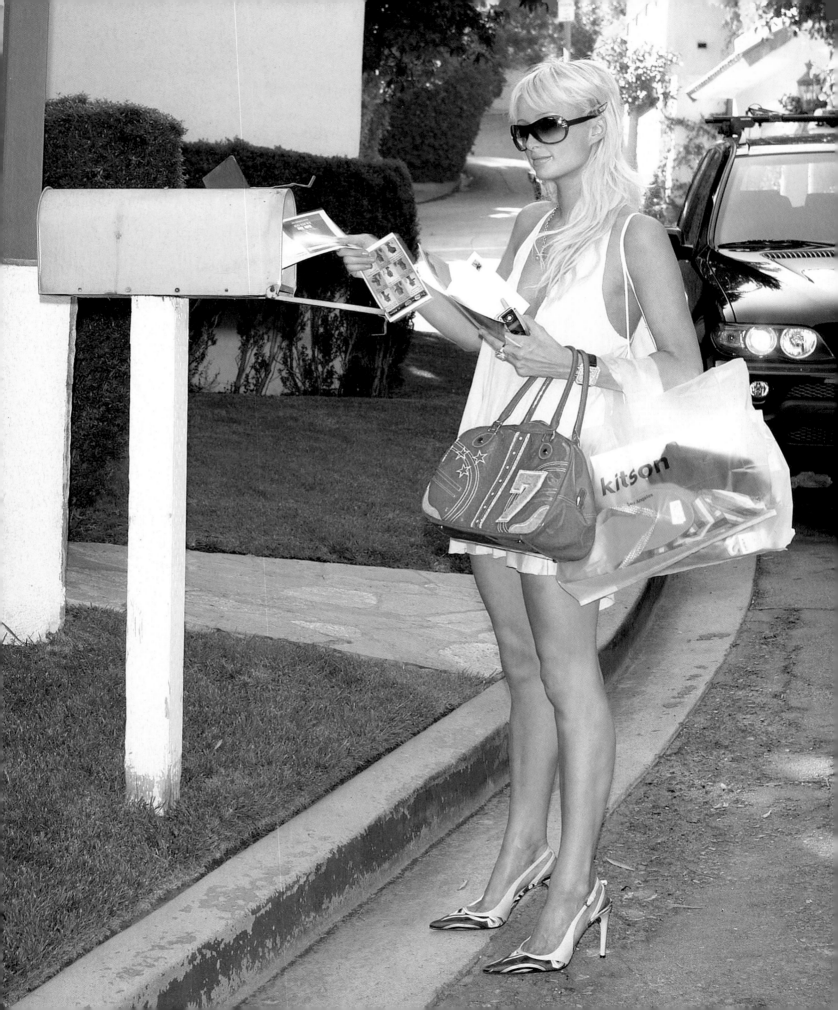

# "ALWAYS BE MORE IMPORTANT THAN YOUR CLOTHES."

—PARIS HILTON, IN A MOMENT OF WISDOM

# PHOTO CREDITS

Tim Rooke/Rex USA. Page 65: Cityfiles/Globe Photos; Nina Prommer/Globe Photos; Brenda Chase/Getty Images. Page 66 (from left): Lucy Nicholson/Reuters/Landov; Riquet/Bauer-Griffin.com; Steve Finn/Getty Images. Page 67 (from left): Sara De Boer/Retna Ltd.; Vince Bucci/Getty Images; Pascal Guyot/AFP/Getty Images; Stephen Trupp/Starmax. Page 68: Eva Sereny/Camera Press/Retna Ltd. Page 69 (clockwise from top): Eva Sereny/Camera Press/Retna Ltd.; Fred Prouser/ Reuters/Landov; Mark Mainz/Getty Images; Gary Lewis/Camera Press Digital/Retna Ltd.; Fairchild Publications; Gregory Pace/Filmmagic.com. Page 71 (clockwise from left): Gilbert Flores/ Celebrityphoto.com; Jeff Vespa/Wireimage.com; Getty Images; Justin Kahn/Wireimage.com; Frederick M. Brown/Getty Images. Page 72 (from left): Courtesy of DVF; Gregory Pace /Filmmagic.com; Chris Polk/Filmmagic.com; Jeff Kravitz/Filmmagic.com. Page 73 (from left): Jill Johnson/JPIstudios.com; Bill Davila/ Filmmagic.com. Page 74–75 (Still Life): Michael Pirrocco/Wenner Media.

CHAPTER 5: Page 77: Michael Germana/UPI/ Landov. Page 78 (from left): INFGoff.com; Arnaldo Magnani/Getty Images; Frederic Nebinger/Abaca. Page 79 (from left): Kevin Winter/Getty Images; Frederick M. Brown/Getty Images (2). Page 80 (from left): Dave Hogan/ Getty Images; Steve Granitz/Wireimage.com; Dave Hogan/Getty Images. Page 81 (from left): Dennis Van Tine/London Features; Sara DeBoer/ Retna Ltd.; Dave Hogan/Getty Images. Page 82: M. Garrett/Getty Images. Page 83 (clockwise from top left): Gene Kornman/MPTV; Henry McGee/Globe Photos; Dave Benett/Getty Images; Matt Campbell/EPA/Sipa Press; MPTV. Page 85 (clockwise from top left): Lawrence Lucier/ Filmmagic.com; Bill Davila/Startraksphoto.com; James Devaney/Wireimage.com; Tsuni/Gamma; Jean-Paul Aussenard/Wireimage.com. Page 86:

Lucy Nicholson/Reuters/Landov. Still Life: Michael Pirrocco/Wenner Media. Page 87 (from left): AP/Wide World Photos; Jeff Haynes/AFP/Getty Images. Pages 88–89 (Still Life): Michael Pirrocco/Wenner Media. Page 91: Michael Caulfield/Wireimage.com.

CHAPTER 6: Page 93 (from left): Arnaldo Magnani/Getty Images; Eric Gaillard/Reuters/ Landov; James Devaney/Wireimage.com; Carlo Allegri/Getty Images. Page 94 (from left): Frederick M. Brown/Getty Images; Ita Mol/Rex USA; Axelle/Bauer-Griffin.com; Mark Sullivan/ Wireimage.com. Page 95 (from left): Anthony Dixon/London Features; Jamie McCarthy/ Wireimage.com; Donato Sardella/ Wireimage.com; Glenn Weiner/Zuma Press. Pages 96–97 (Still Life): Michael Pirrocco/ Wenner Media.

CHAPTER 7: Page 101: Bill Davila/ Startraksphoto.com. Page 102 (from left): Ginsburg-Spaly/X17agency.com; Lawrence Schwartzwald/Splashnews.com. Page 103 (from left): Boldeskul/Vaughan/ACE Pictures; Mark Calleja/Alpha/Globe Photos. Page 104: Avik Gilboa/Wireimage.com (2). Page 105 (from left): Donato Sardella/Wireimage.com; Fame Pictures. Page 106 (from left): Steve Granitz/ Wireimage.com; Jeff Vespa/Wireimage.com. Page 107 (from left): Michael Rozman/ Filmmagic.com; Splashnews.com. Page 108 (from left): Jeffrey Mayer/Wireimage.com; Camilla Morandi/Rex USA. Page 109 (from left): Jeffrey Mayer/Wireimage.com; INFGoff.com. Page 110: John Kobal Foundation/Getty Images. Page 111: Studio Patellani/Corbis. Pages 110–111 (Still Life): Michael Pirrocco/Wenner Media. Page 112: Douglas Miller/ Getty Images. Page 113: Art Rickerby/Time Life Pictures/Getty Images. Pages 112–113 (Still Life): Michael Pirrocco/Wenner Media. Page 115: Lawrence Schwartzwald/Splashnews.com.

CHAPTER 8: Page 117: Mark Mainz/Getty Images. Page 118 (from left): Nancy Kaszerman/ Zuma Press; Chris Polk/Filmmagic.com. Page 119 (from left): Stewart Cook/Rex USA; Albert L. Ortega/Wireimage.com. Page 120 (clockwise from top left): Dennis Van Tine/London Features; Jen Lowery/London Features; Michael Williams/London Features; Mark Mainz/Getty Images; Ray Mickshaw/Wireimage.com; Jen Lowery/London Features; John Sciulli/Wireimage.com; AP/Wide World Photos. Page 121 (clockwise from top left): Jemal Countess/Wireimage.com; Lawrence Lucier/Filmmagic.com; Paul Cooper/Rex USA; Lisa Rose/JPIstudios.com; Zak Brian/Gamma; Jon Kopaloff/Filmmagic.com; Gregory Pace/ Filmmagic.com; Lisa Rose/JPIstudios.com. Page 122 (from left): Axelle/Bauer-Griffin.com; Erik C. Pendzich/Rex USA. Page 123 (from left): Gregg DeGuire/Wireimage.com; Lionel Hahn/ ABACA. Page 124 (from left): Andrea Renault/ Globe Photos; Steve Kondiles/Bauer-Griffin.com. Page 125 (from left): Jean-Paul Aussenard/ Wireimage.com; Tom Rodriguez/Globe Photos. Page 126 (from left): Mike Marsland/ Wireimage.com; Jim Spellman/Wireimage.com. Page 127 (from left): James Devaney/ Wireimage.com; Axelle/Bauer-Griffin.com. Page 128: Steve Granitz/Wireimage.com. Page 129 (from top): James Devaney/Wireimage.com; Jeff Kravitz/Filmmagic.com; Jean-Paul Aussenard/Wireimage.com. Pages 128–129 (Still Life): Michael Pirrocco/Wenner Media. Page 131: Stewart Cook/Rex USA.

CHAPTER 9: Page 133: Richard Young/Rex USA. Page 134 (from left): Vince Bucci/Getty Images; Gregory Pace/Filmmagic.com. Page 135 (from left): Paul Fenton/KPA/Keystone Pictures/Zuma Press; Kathy Hutchins/Hutchins Photo Agency. Page 136 (from left): Jeff Vespa/Wireimage.com; James Devaney/Wireimage.com. Page 137 (from left): Jim Smeal/BEImages.net; Colin Knight/

JPIstudios.com. Page 138 (from left): Dimitrios Kambouris/Wireimage.com; Henry McGee/ Globe Photos. Page 139 (from left): Carlo Allegri/Getty Images; Gilbert Flores/ Celebrityphoto.com. Pages 140-141 (Still Life): Michael Pirrocco/Wenner Media. Page 142: Mike Blake/Reuters/Landov. Page 143 (from left): Eric Gaillard/ Reuters/Landov; Dave Benett/Getty Images.

Page 144 (from left): Paolo Pirez/LMK/Photolink; AP/Wide World Photos. Page 145: Peter Brooker/ Rex USA. Page 146: Chris Delmas/Zuma Press. Page 147 (from left): Russell Einhorn/ Splashnews.com; Francis Specker/Landov. Page 148 (from left): Niviere/Aslan/Villard/Sipa Press; Jim Smeal/Wireimage.com. Page 149: Jeff Kravitz/Filmmagic.com.

CHAPTER 10: Page 153: Chris Delmas/ VISUALPressAgency.com. Page 154 (from left): Gregory Pace/Filmmagic.com; Newsmakers/ Getty Images. Page 155 (clockwise from top left): Sara De Boer/Retna Ltd.; Tsuni/Gamma; Matthew Peyton/Getty Images; Lisa Rose/ JPIstudios.com; Dimitrios Kambouris/ Wireimage.com; Jean Baptiste Lacroix/ Wireimage.com; Gregory Pace/Filmmagic.com; Rex USA. Page 156 (from left): Hahn/Khayat/ ABACA; Frederick M. Brown/Getty Images. Page 157 (clockwise from top left): Vince Bucci/Getty Images; Jon Kopaloff/ Filmmagic.com; Lawrence Lucier/Getty Images; Frederic Nebinger/ABACA; Evan Agostini/Getty Images; Nicolas Khayat/ ABACA; Jeffrey Mayer/ Wireimage.com; Tony Barson/Wireimage.com. Page 158 (from left): Lawrence Lucier/Getty Images; SR066/ZBP/Zuma Press. Page 159 (clockwise from top left): Walter Weissman/Starmax; Theo Wargo/ Wireimage.com; Jen Lowery/London Features; Richard C. Murray/London Features; Lionel Hahn/ABACA; Kevin Mazur/ Wireimage.com; Jim Smeal/Wireimage.com; Axelle/Bauer-Griffin.com. Page 160 (from left): Bill Davila/

Filmmagic.com; Myung Jung Kim/ PA/ABACA. Page 161 (clockwise from top left): Erik C. Pendzich/Rex USA; Patrick Rideaux/Rex USA; Kevin Winter/Getty Images; Lawrence Lucier/ Getty Images; Francis Specker/EPA/Landov; Chris Polk/Filmmagic.com; Frederick M. Brown/Getty Images; Fitzroy Barrett/Globe Photos. Page 162 (from left): Evan Agostini/Getty Images; Jennifer Graylock/JPIstudios.com. Page 163 (clockwise from top left): J. Scott Wynn/Retna Ltd.; Milan Ryba/Globe Photos; Steve Granitz/ Wireimage.com; Adam Nemser/Photolink; Barry Talesnick/IPOL/Globe Photos; Lawrence Schwartzwald/Splashnews.com; Ron Galella/ Wireimage.com; XLNY/London Features. Page 164: Tsuni/Gamma.

CHAPTER 11: Page 167: Matrix/Bauer-Griffin.com. Page 168 (from left): N. Warren Winter/Zuma Press; AS001/GS001/ZBP/Zuma Press. Page 169 (from left): No Credit; Arnaldo Magnani/Getty Images; Lucky Mat/Getty Images. Page 170 (from left): Carlo Allegri/Getty Images; John Barrett/Globe Photos. Page 171 (from left): Jim Spellman/Wireimage.com; Tom Kingston/ Wireimage.com; Chris Polk/Filmmagic.com. Page 172 (from left): Piel Patrick/Gamma; Dennis Van Tine/London Features; Richard Chambury/Globe Photos. Page 173 (from left): Ramey Photo Agency; Ethan Miller/Reuters/ Landov; Matrix/Bauer-Griffin.com. Page 174 (from left): Avik Gilboa/Wireimage.com; Nancy Kaszerman/Zuma Press; Jeff Vespa/ Wireimage.com. Page 175 (from left): Flynetpictures.com; Ramey Photo Agency; Venturelli/Romaniello/Olympia/Sipa Press.
Page 177: Brian Snyder/Reuters/Landov.

CHAPTER 12: Page 179: Anthony Phelps/Reuters/Landov. Page 180, from left: Amy Graves/Wireimage.com; Fernando Allende/Celebrityphoto.com. Page 181 (clock-

wise from top left): Bill Davila/Filmmagic.com; Tsuni/Gamma; Jen Lowery/London Features; Dennis Van Tine/London Features; Jen Lowery/London Features; Eric Ryan/Getty Images; Axelle/Bauer-Griffin.com; Jill Johnson/ JPIstudios.com. Page 182 (from left): Jean-Paul Aussenard/Wireimage.com; Michael Williams/ London Features. Page 183 (clockwise from top left): Ed Geller/Globe Photos; Henry McGee/ Globe Photos; Jemal Countess/Wireimage.com; Steve Granitz/Wireimage.com; Randy Brooke/ Wireimage.com; Jeff Kravitz/Filmmagic.com; Paul Fenton/KPA/Keystone Pictures/Zuma Press; Lawrence Lucier/Filmmagic.com. Page 184 (from left): Roger Wong/INF/Starmax; Jim Ruymen/Reuters/Landov. Page 185 (clockwise

## Answers to Sunglasses Quiz
PAGES 16-17:

1. Anna Nicole Smith
2. Elizabeth Taylor
3. Marisa Tomei
4. Natalie Wood
5. Sarah Jessica Parker
6. Charlize Theron
7. Jennifer Lopez
8. Sophia Loren
9. Christina Applegate
10. Grace Kelly
11. Scarlett Johansson
12. Alicia Keys
13. Diana Ross
14. Paris Hilton
15. Beyoncé Knowles
16. Drew Barrymore
17. Catherine Deneuve
18. Nicole Kidman
19. Doris Day
20. Selma Blair
21. Gwen Stefani
22. Lindsay Lohan
23. Audrey Hepburn
24. Jessica Simpson

from top left): Roger Wong/INF/Starmax; Jon Kopaloff/Filmmagic.com; UMDADC/Rex USA; Jean Catuffe/Sipa Press; Splashnews.com; Amy Graves/Globe Photos; Steve Butler/Sipa Press; SR066/ZBP/Zuma Press. Page 186 (from left): Andrea Renault/Globe Photos; Lisa Rose/JPIstudios.com. Page 187 (clockwise from top left): NYPP/Zuma Press; Shelly Doss/JPIstudios.com; Frank Trapper/Corbis; Ed Geller/Globe Photos; Gregory Pace/Filmmagic.com; David Buchan/Rex USA; Kevin Mazur/Wireimage.com; Richard Orjis/PMC/Sipa Press. Page 188: Chris Weeks/Wireimage.com.

CHAPTER 13: Page 191: Lionel Hahn/ABACA. Page 192 (from left): Robin Platzer/Filmmagic.com; Jennifer Graylock/JPIstudios.com; Mark Larkin/London Features. Page 193: Trevor Kent/INFGoff.com. Page 194 (from left): WENN/Landov; Gregory Pace/Filmmagic.com; Jay Thornton/INFGoff.com. Page 195: Blanco-Ginsburg/X17agency.com. Page 196 (from left): George Pimentel/Wireimage.com; Jean-Paul Aussenard/Wireimage.com; JA501/ZBP/Zuma Press. Page 197: Jon Kopaloff/Filmmagic.com. Page 198 (from left): LDP Images; Jonathan Friolo/IHP/Splashnews.com; Frank Trapper/Corbis. Page 199: RE/Westcom Image/ABACA. Page 200: Frank Micelotta/Getty Images. Page 201: Theo Wargo/Wireimage.com. Page 202: Lionel Hahn/ABACA. Page 203: Lawrence Lucier/Filmmagic.com. Still Life: Michael Pirrocco/Wenner Media.

CHAPTER 14: Page 205: Stephane Cardinale/Corbis. Page 206 (from left): Gilbert Flores/Celebrityphoto.com, Gregory Pace/Filmmagic.com. Page 207 (clockwise from top left): Paul Hawthorne/Wireimage.com; Erik C. Pendzich/Rex USA; Jason Merritt/Filmmagic.com; Gregory Pace/Filmmagic.com; Fernando Allende/Celebrityphoto.com; Frank Trapper/Corbis; Jennifer Graylock/JPIstudios.com; Dimitrios

Kambouris/Wireimage.com. Page 208 (from left): Dennis Van Tine/London Features; Rota/PA/ABACA. Page 209 (clockwise from top left): Jen Lowery/London Features; Dave Allocca/Startraksphoto.com; Kevin Mazur/Wireimage.com; Jennifer Graylock/JPIstudios.com; SSO01/ZBP/Zuma Press; Carmen Valdes/Retna Ltd.; Lawrence Schwartzwald/Splashnews.com; ACE005/ACE Pictures. Page 210 (from left): Djamilla Rosa Cochran/Wireimage.com; Gregg DeGuire/Wireimage.com. Page 211 (clockwise from top left): Oliver Polter/Alpha/Globe Photos; Kathy Hutchins/Hutchins Photo; Anthony Dixon/London Features; Matrix/Bauer-Griffin.com; Kevin Mazur/Wireimage.com; Ramey Photo Agency; Gregg DeGuire/Wireimage.com; Nina Prommer/Globe Photos. Page 212 (from left): Robert Galbraith/Reuters/Landov; Fitzroy Barrett/Globe Photos. Page 213 (clockwise from top left): John Schults/Reuters/Corbis; James Devaney/Wireimage.com; Dave Benett/Getty Images; James Devaney/Wireimage.com; Jeff Vespa/Wireimage.com; Jeff Snyder/Filmmagic.com; Lisa O'Connor/Zuma Press; Frank Trapper/Corbis. Page 214 (from left): Russ Einhorn/Starmax; James Devaney/Wireimage.com. Page 215 (clockwise from top left): Mario Anzuoni/Splashnews.com; Jon Kopaloff/Filmmagic.com; Fitzroy Barrett/Globe Photos; Nils Jorgensen/Rex USA; Lawrence Lucier/Filmmagic.com; Lisa Rose/JPIstudios.com; Bill Davila/Filmmagic.com; Ramey Photo Agency. Page 216: Ramey Photo Agency.

## ADDITIONAL FASHION CREDITS

Page 96: (left) dress, Talbots; earrings, Banana Republic; watch, Gucci; bag, Elaine Turner; scarf, Banana Republic; shoes, Ann Taylor LOFT; (right) hat, Nine West; necklace, Jules NY; bag, Ipa-Nima; shoes, Francesca Giobbi

Page 97: (left) earrings, Tommy Hilfiger; clutch, Franchi; watch, Rolex; boots, Stuart Weitzman; (right) star earrings, Mia & Kompany; fur shrug, Shin Choi; brooch on shrug, Carol Dauplaise; gloves, La Crasia; bag, Valentino; shoes, Valentino

Page 110: white tie-top, Kulson; shorts, Tracy Reese, earrings, Givenchy; bag, Tocca; shoes, C. Ronson

Page 111: dress, ABS by Allen Schwartz; headscarf, Adrienne Vittadini; bag, Dooney & Bourke; boots, Coach

Page 112: button-down shirt, Theory; jacket, Tommy Jeans; trousers, Express; brooch, RJ Graziano; bag, Kooba; snakeskin pumps, Luisa Beccaria

Page 113: dress, Milly; bracelet, H by Tommy Hilfiger; sunglasses, Oliver Peoples; bag, Banana Republic; sandals, Jack Rogers

Page 140: (left) sequined top, Hidy Ng; pants, Theory; earrings and ring, M&J Savitt; shoes, Rickard Shah; (right) dress, BCBG; earrings, Erickson Beamon; clutch, Clara Kasavina; shoes, Hollywould

Page 141: (left) skirt, jacket, and bustier, Monique Lhuillier; earrings, Mia & Kompany; clutch, Judith Leiber; shoes, Sergio Rossi; (right) gown, Alberta Ferretti; bracelet, Jules NY; bag, Tods; shoes, Pollini

# INDEX